SPANDEX NOT COMPULSORY

How to Get (and Remain) Strong, Fit and Confident without Restrictive Rules

JOONAS HEIKKINEN

Foreword by Chris Vein

SPANDEX NOT COMPULSORY
How to Get (and Remain) Strong, Fit and Confident
without Restrictive Rules

Joonas Heikkinen

Foreword by Chris Vein

Copyright © 2018 Joonas Heikkinen

Foreword © 2018 Chris Vein

Published by Full View Publishing

Edited by Jessica Hoadley

Book format design by Eled Cernik

Cover design by Predrag Capo

Paperback ISBN 978-0-646-98655-5
eBook ISBN 978-0-646-98656-2

Disclaimer

The author of this material is not responsible in any manner for any injury that may occur through following the instructions contained in this material. The activities, physical and otherwise, contained in this book are for informational use only and should not be considered as medical advice, diagnosis or treatment. Readers should seek advice from their healthcare provider before starting any exercise or diet program.

To Colleen,

For all the love, grace and patience

TABLE OF CONTENTS

FOREWORD

"Thank you for giving me my life back."

Sounds a bit melodramatic doesn't it? But not for me.

At age 35, I had my first back surgery. At age 45, I had my second and third. My fourth back surgery that same year was to implant electrodes along my spine to trick my brain into not feeling pain. It didn't work. Neither did the myriad of pain management drug cocktails my pain doctor prescribed. At age 46, I said enough and went cold turkey. No more drugs. I vowed to manage my pain by recognising it, putting it in a box, moving it aside, and focusing on living my life. It worked. But at the cost of energy taken from other parts of the body.

These were also the years of climbing the corporate ladder. Leading technology for a major US city, attempting the same for the whole US government in the White House, and then, working to eradicate extreme poverty across the globe through an international development organisation. I was never home, which created an incredible amount of stress on my marriage. I travelled a lot – one year, I flew over 340,000 miles. My diet was poor. And I was sleep-deprived, falling asleep in elevators, restaurants, taxis.

Fast forward five years and I was still living in the US but commuting to Sydney where I was building a new global consulting practice. I was noticeably limping and starting to hunch over when I walked. I was scared. I knew I needed help. Fast.

A new gym opened very near where I lived and worked. The gym's sales guy asked what I was looking for in a trainer. After listening a bit, he had that aha moment and said, "Have I got the guy for you". And thus, began my life changing experience with Joonas Heikkinen (or Mr H for those of us not from Finland).

Giving me my life back proved to be frustratingly slow. At three months, I had relearned how to crawl. Seriously. Do you know how humbling it is to be in the middle of a gym as a middle-aged guy trying to crawl?

Fast forward one year and I'm a new person. Well, I feel like one anyway. My chronic pain is reduced. I walk as I'm supposed to. Straight. I don't limp. My body fat has dropped. And my energy levels are through the roof.

I'm jealous of those who read this book – I had to learn it over time through challenging, and at times, frustrating training sessions. You get to read it, although you do miss out on hearing him talk endlessly about his cats and heavy metal bands. But I digress. He taught me, and will teach you too through this book, three major lessons:

1. Training should focus on making one better at living. I rebelled. I will be honest. *Spandex Not Compulsory* asks about goals, what is important, what isn't. Hell, all I wanted at first was to be able to crawl and not look like an idiot. But over time, the process outlined in this book led me on a journey of self-discovery. Once I understood why I wanted what I wanted and how much I was willing to give up to get my way, my mindset shifted. This time was different to years before when I was solely focused on looking better and paid a large price by blowing

out my right knee. Sure, I still wanted my six-pack. I still wanted bigger legs. But this time, rather than focus on illusive gains, I learned to focus on how my six-pack and bigger legs would help me achieve my broader life goals – something as basic as providing the physical foundation to survive all that life threw at me. It is empowering in its simplicity.

2. Training should be about learning the skills behind the method. "First move well and then move often" is a quote in this book and it also defines *Spandex Not Compulsory*. This is frustrating; well, it was for me. I only wanted to bench press and squat. Instead I was learning how to crawl, walk, carry kettlebells, slam balls and stretch. I wanted to tear my hair out. But Joonas has a patient and persistent approach. It won me over. I've always known I should focus on form, but Joonas taught me why and how to do it. And yes, I did bench press and squat too.

3. You cannot out-train an unhealthy diet. I come from a farming background where generations before me had been fantastic cooks. But they cooked for people who did physical labour 24 hours a day, 365 days a year. And sugar was part of every meal. Again, I knew what I was supposed to do, but I could never do it consistently. So, I would lift more weights, do more reps, go to the gym more often. I lost body fat but also lost muscle. The approach outlined in *Spandex Not Compulsory* taught me that my diet and recovery are as important as the time I spend in the gym.

This is a thinking person's book. It doesn't provide an easy way out of the mental, physical, and emotional challenges of training. It doesn't promise fast weight loss or rapid muscle gain. Frankly, I wish it did, but I know now that those promises are empty.

Spandex Not Compulsory is about taking control – owning one's life. And owning one's health is simply the only way to do that. Following the principles in this book requires persistence. But it isn't judgemental. It lets us be human and supports us when we really screw up. And we will. Constantly. However, this approach asks us to identify what we want and the price we are willing to pay. "Extremely simple, yet frustratingly difficult" cannot be truer. But the payoff is huge.

I call *Spandex Not Compulsory* the gospel according to Joonas. Believe in it and it will change your life. It did for me.

Chris Vein

PREFACE

The Story of a Recovering Fitness Addict

There's a personal reason why I preach about a *reasonable* approach to health and fitness: at times, my relationship with fitness has been anything but. I remember travelling to Sydney for the time in 2005 and training on most days when my buddies went to do what other travellers do: relax on the beach, drink coffee and zone out with cheap wine. I should've been enjoying the warm summer days exploring the new city, but I decided to spend most of the trip doing bicep curls. I couldn't justify enjoying myself unless I got the training in.

Fast forward two years to 2007 and I was training four to seven times a week, close to two hours at a time. Everything I ate or drank was based on how much I would have to train to burn off the calories. No matter how much I trained, I was never happy with how I looked. By then, I was getting compliments from people saying that I looked great. Compliments acted like gasoline to fire – they fed my obsession. At that point, I was already well on my way to becoming orthorexic (an eating disorder that involves taking one's healthy eating to an extreme). I was counting calories, and only choosing the "purest" of foods. Food selection became a moral choice; it was either "good" or "bad" for me.

Eating and training became a religion, and I devoted all my time to worshipping the unholy lord of fitness.

Then I took my first personal training job in a gym that was full of bodybuilders. Their definition of letting loose on a Saturday night was putting a tablespoon of low-sodium tomato sauce on a chicken breast. If it wasn't already, life now became all about how you looked, and that's how I judged the value of myself and others.

My life had no balance whatsoever: my wife (girlfriend at the time) must've thought that she'd lost her partner to the "health" industry. I put health in quotes because, as you can tell, none of the actions I took made me any healthier. I thought that if I wanted to have a career in the fitness industry, this was how my life had to be.

I was constantly getting sick because I wasn't eating the wide variety of foods that a well-functioning body needs. But I was not able to connect the dots between my actions and how I felt. I avoided going out because of how it would affect my looks – eating out required letting go of control. Eating was not enjoyable, it was more like a maths class of counting calories. Food was not fun; it was purely consumed for fuel. It wasn't about flavours but protein, fats and carbs. If I didn't eat from a (home-prepared) Tupperware container, I would freak out because I had no idea what sort of evil intruders would invade my body. I know this sounds nuts, but I was so immersed in the situation I couldn't see the fingers from the fist.

Living a life using fitness as the only guiding value is not fun. Yet I thought I was doing everything right. And, like most people who take fitness to the extremes, I thought I was at the pinnacle of health. Looking back now, I see that I was lacking self-confidence, and was compensating for it by making myself look as good as possible.

I still remember the moment I realised I had a problem. That maybe I was not juggling all the balls at the same time. I went to the grocery store with a friend. He picked up a roasted chicken, and I grabbed a packet of rice crackers. I weighed all of 77 kg at the time (I am just shy of 190 cm tall, on a good day). His exact words were "Dude, you shop like you're trying to lose weight". It dropped like a sledgehammer in my forehead. The difference was that this came from a peer who was in better shape than I was, yet he still seemed to enjoy more things in life than just training. After that moment, little by little, I became more aware of what was going on. It was a gradual shift in thinking.

When you are new at something and still finding your feet, many of your actions are based on those around you. When I started taking health and training more seriously, I thought the only reason to do it was to look like a fitness model. After years of this mindset, I was gradually able to shift my values to health and strength and aesthetics, instead of only aesthetics. I found what feels right for me. I discovered what I value in life and based my actions on those values.

INTRODUCTION

Every one of us wants to be fit, strong and healthy, and feel confident about our body. But not everybody wants, or needs, to be an athlete, a powerlifter, bodybuilder, or a lycra-wearing fitness addict. Most people don't have the time or the interest for any of that. And that's normal. This book is for normal people. It's not a quick fix or a fad. It doesn't focus on a one-size-fits-all technical program or diet. Instead, it gives you the principles for a sustainable approach to fitness – an approach that you'll be able to continue, no matter what life throws your way.

Maybe you are desperate to improve your health and fitness, but limited by time or enthusiasm? Maybe you are stuck on a road to nowhere jumping from one fad to the next, trying to figure out how to stay motivated to use that gym membership you signed up for? Or maybe you are confused and frustrated about all the health and fitness hype on the internet, where one piece of advice seems to contradict the next. After all, you can go to Google, type in any health or fitness goal your heart desires and get a solid thousand ways to accomplish that goal, give or take a few. If your health and fitness could be measured by the abundance of information available today, you should be fit enough to cross any of the great seven seas with a casual afternoon swim.

The downside of a free flow of information is that too much noise paralyses you from acting on the information that matters. The noise can lead you to believe that the next sexy fad diet and hardcore training plan is better than the one you are currently on. Now – hold on to your seat here – I propose that you don't need sexy fad diets and hardcore training plans to get this done. *Gasp! Shock! Horror! Mephistopheles of all thing sacred in fitness!*

There's a sweet spot within fitness, training and healthy eating. Too far in any one direction pushes life out of balance. I want you to discover and spend the rest of your life in that sweet spot when it comes to fitness. The word I am looking for is *reasonable*, as sexy as it sounds.

This book will help you get awesome at the basics. Basics are rather simple but not necessarily easy. There are no shortcuts or magic tricks. This will require a lot of hard work on your end, and at times there are no clear rules to follow. You will have to do some soul-searching and it will be uncomfortable. But persevere and you'll learn a great deal about yourself along the way. In the end it will be all worth the effort – you will become the master of your own body. You will learn what works for you.

Fitness should be something that adds value and quality to your life. It should allow you to live a louder, richer, more energetic life outside of the gym. Strength coach extraordinaire Dan John has a saying, "Fitness is an ability to do a task". For us this means: don't train and exercise because you want to be better at training and exercising. Train and exercise because you want to be better at life.

I honestly think that a life spent chasing the perfect body is a life wasted. It'll never be enough, and you'll miss a lot of great moments while doing so. Do you want to be on your deathbed listening to people talk about how jacked you looked in the summer of 2018? Or do you want them to talk about how happy you made them feel?

Not wearing spandex and being reasonable with fitness is not a hall pass to ignore your health. It's about finding a balance – finding your *reasonable*. Pursue things that make you feel content, even happy, while being a positive influence in other people's lives: your newly found fitness and energy will give you more presence and vigour than ever before. You and the people close to you deserve it.

Before you go further, there are writing assignments for you to do throughout this book. To make the book more useful, I've included a free bonus workbook. You can download it at **RepsAndTheRest.com/ SpandexNotCompulsory**

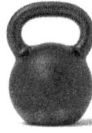

PART 1

In The Beginning...

ESCAPING THE MIND JAIL

Your mindset plays a big, and often ignored, part in your ability to achieve goals – whether it's in fitness and health, or life in general. When you are facing an uncomfortable situation and don't believe that you can do it, you are making things harder for yourself before you even get started. It's not that positive thinking magically manifests in positive results. I am not going drown you in pseudoscience by telling you that to compete in ski jump for your country at the next Olympics all you must do is believe, hard (cue "I believe I can fly" by R. Kelly here). Rather, positive thinking can lead you to slowly changing your everyday psychology, the way you approach life and the challenges it brings. A positive approach to life can lead you to make better decisions in the long term. What's more, there is research on optimism and how it's robustly associated with a lower risk of mortality.

You might be going through that right now. In which case (talk about a great timing), when facing an uncomfortable situation, I like to ask myself two questions:

1. What is the worst thing that can happen?

Unless I am planning a stunt à la Evel Knievel, the worst possible outcome is most likely *not* earth (or bone) shattering.

2. If I bomb, will any of this matter in 10 years?

If the answer is a resounding *no,* why worry about it? This is something I use every time before getting on stage for an improv theatre show. And as someone who often catastrophises things in my head, this little thought exercise helps me to rationalise them. It helps me to form a sort of *come whatever may* attitude while holding on to a *get out of jail free* card.

Bringing this back to fitness, when you load up a heavy deadlift, provided that it's not an absurd amount of weight for you, but keep telling yourself that there's no chance of it leaving the ground, guess what? It probably won't leave the ground. It's not because your beliefs miraculously affected your physical capabilities. It's because your negative attitude about the lift made you stop before you gave it 110% effort. If that's what you choose to do, you might as well go home, sit on the couch and play *Mario Kart.*

When you think that there is no chance you can go a week without drinking wine, you are probably right. It's likely that you'll fall flat on your face (into the wine glass) when you see yourself failing at something before even giving it a proper go. Your physical actions will gravitate towards what your mind believes. The connection between the body and the mind is like a firm handshake between old friends.

This is not magic

Just because there's a mind–body connection doesn't mean that you should become overly optimistic about everything. You won't grow rich or bend forks with your brainpower just by believing it can happen. You can't use "earthling" (thanks, celebrity "health gurus") as a substitute for eating a bowl of porridge. Believing, no matter how hard you do it, doesn't materialise in things that are unrealistic, at best. But you know that already. What believing can do, though, is get you a positive outcome in a tight situation. The template for being successful in this health and fitness thing is to prepare, keep practising and learning while doing so, and have a *yes, I can do this* mindset. If one of those things is missing, the road ahead is going to be harder than it needs to be.

SELF–SHAMING IS CORRODING YOUR CHANCES OF CHANGE

After reading *Daring Greatly: How the Courage to Be Vulnerable Transforms the Way We Live, Love, Parent, and Lead* by Brené Brown, I started to pay attention to how much people talk themselves down. And since I spend most of my time training clients in a gym, this negative self-talk is most often related to one's body and self-image.

"I am fat." "I am so weak." "I am bad at this." "I can't do this." I hear these statements every day. Brown calls this "shame-talk" and it has negative consequences on your self-worth and wellbeing, and to your chances of succeeding.

Think how you would feel if your friend told you each day what a failure you are or how fat you are – or how much you suck at life in general. This is what self-blaming shame-talk is: you are telling yourself that you are not worth it, that you are not good enough. You might use shame as motivation, thinking that it's what pushes you to conquer your goals. Yet accordingly to Brown, "Researchers don't find shame correlated with positive outcomes at all" and, "There are no data to support that shame is a helpful compass for good behavior". Shame is more likely to be the catalyst of destructive and hurtful behaviour than be part of the solution.

Shame vs guilt

Shame relates to self and says, "I am bad". It is highly correlated with addiction, depression and eating disorders, among other health issues. It keeps us small, resentful and afraid. Shame can also make us rationalise or blame our actions on others: I ate a family-size tub of ice-cream because "it was Friday", "I was stressed", "my friend didn't like my singing", "it was a full moon". Shame will try to justify the actions we take.

However, when we accept and take ownership of our actions, guilt, rather than shame, is usually the driving force. Guilt relates to actions, and says, "I did something bad". And no matter how uncomfortable guilt feels, it can also be helpful: psychological discomfort can motivate a meaningful change. Guilt's influence is positive, unlike shame, which is destructive. Brown explains that shame corrodes the belief that we can change and do better. Not a very good long-term motivator, is it?

When it comes to shame-talk, I find this advice about cultivating self-compassion while letting go of perfectionism from Brown especially important: "Healthy striving is self-focused: How can I improve? Perfectionism is other-focused: What will they think?"

As long as your actions align with your values (we'll go into this later), you've got nothing to be ashamed of. The troubles start once you let others guide your actions. I guess it's partly about not giving a shit about what other people think about you. Provided that you are not being an obnoxious and arrogant brat. But that's a given.

To escape your own mind jail, you need to cultivate positive thinking, take action, and not be weighed down by destructive feelings of shame.

WHY IS HEALTH AND FITNESS CONFUSING?

Often we get ourselves pigeonholed into a strict, biased camp of a certain approach to fitness. I am the first to put my hand up and say that I'm guilty of that, too. We end up treating our diet and training methods as a religion. But out of all the fitness celebrities and diet book authors in the world, who has the right answer? Well, it depends on what you enjoy doing. You should do whatever gets you moving while keeping you healthy. Vague? That's sort of the point.

You have to experiment with what's right for you for the long term. Despite what the most recent science (or advertising) might say is the "best" diet and fitness regime, it is useless for you if you can't follow it. Whatever it is that you decide to follow, here's a principle to use as your guiding light: *Does this get me to where I want to go by the safest, most sustainable way possible?*

Pick up any reasonably sane diet book in the bookshop and they usually have a few things in common: eat four serves of protein a day, plenty of vegetables, focus mostly on wholefoods and don't drink your calories. At most times, those recommendations work for most people. Those with specific conditions, goals or certain illnesses might need the super-specific, special and advanced high-carb, low-carb, high-fat, low-fat, only eat during the high tide, only use one chopstick while eating a soup diet, and so on. That is beyond this book and my scope of practice. If you follow the basic principles for three months (most people don't) and don't see results, it might be time to consult a dietitian.

But what often happens is that when one of these super-specific, special and advanced diets works for a certain group of people, they go on morning television to talk about it, and then everyone starts doing it. If one of these diet followers is a celebrity, this is how a new diet cult/religion is born. Once again, we've made something very simple into something more complicated than it has to be.

Stick to basics and keep it simple. Stop chasing all things new and shiny. Don't try to force a square peg into a round hole. Don't follow the herd to the latest magic solution. Step aside and observe and you'll notice over time how this same cycle repeats itself over and over again. Each time, it seems we've learned nothing.

If something doesn't feel right, it probably isn't right for you. However, just because it feels challenging doesn't mean it's not right. If you've lived your life so far eating cornflakes for breakfast, lunch and dinner, moving away from this habit will be hard. The magic solution? Hard work, dedication and surrounding yourself with supportive and like-minded people.

We all think we are the special snowflakes who need special approaches. Fortunately, it's rarely the case. Don't worry about the super-specific, special and advanced diet information until you've thoroughly tried the simple stuff and gotten as far as you can go. I went from simple to complicated and back to simple because it just worked better.

Focus on the basics. Most of the other stuff is just fluff. And it's this fluff that the diet industry and the marketers thrive on. Maybe I am cynical, but there's a lot of money to be made when people are unhappy and vulnerable to the deception of a "miracle cure".

STRIVING FOR PERFECTION VS BEING PRESENT

Too often we set ourselves major "end goals" in training, weight loss, career and life, and focus solely on getting to that place, wherever it might be. We want to live in that perfect house, earn a certain amount of money, get to a certain weight and reach a certain body fat percentage ... It's the same cycle over and over again: "Once I get to [insert any goal anyone has ever had] it will be perfect, then I will be happy".

Maybe this next analogy reveals the decade in which I was a teenager, but what the hell. To me, this "end goal" chasing resembles the worm game on old Nokia mobile phones: you promise yourself that once you get to 100 points, which meant that the worm had to eat 100 apples without crashing into walls or itself (the tail kept growing with each apple it ate), you'll be done playing. But once you got to 100 points, the target of "enough" moved to 150 points, and so on. It was a never-ending vicious cycle. I spent a lot of my youth chasing those digital apples on the screen.

Once you get to your ultimate goal of perfection it doesn't necessarily feel as extraordinary as you thought it would. So you set yourself another goal and start the same process again: "Once I get to [insert any goal anyone has ever had] it will be perfect, then I will be happy".

We think that if we keep grinding away, we will eventually reach some sort of magical place of perfection. What we forget is to appreciate *now* and where we are at this very moment. Some people live their whole lives trying to get somewhere, never pausing to appreciate how good everything is just at this very moment. Those people are never truly satisfied with what they have as they always feel like their life is missing something – that magic ingredient that would make everything *just perfect.*

It is important for your health to stop at least once a day and just appreciate what you've got. Learn to be happy where you are. Think about how good things are instead of what's wrong or what's missing. So you might not be down to 10% body fat, but how much different would your life actually be if you got there? This doesn't mean that you should stop setting goals and just give up on life. Quite the opposite: constant self-improvement is crucial (if at times overdone in our current world of me, me, me). But don't fall into the trap of thinking that once you get to your goals, life will be perfect or that you will feel as if this is enough.

Forget what other people think of as ideal and what the universal standards for being successful are: how you should look, what weight you should be, what body fat you should attain. These are all external motivators. Don't live your life trying to impress other people but instead seek internal happiness. Are you doing something to live up to someone else's standards? Is society telling you how your life has to be in order to be successful and happy? Are the health and fitness magazines telling you how you should look?

I want you to take a moment to ponder when you will feel satisfied. Have you set your sights on climbing a mountain, thinking that once you get there your life will be perfect? Is it another degree, that promotion, dropping the last three kilograms? Keep in mind that once you get to that mountaintop, there will be another higher mountain behind it, and another behind that. And it is fine to keep climbing them, but don't think that there will be some special moment when you will have climbed enough mountains and reached that ultimate peak.

That moment will never arrive unless you consciously start focusing on being content with what you've got, how you look and how your life is, right at this very moment.

In the beginning, the health and fitness landscape can seem confusing and overwhelming. It doesn't have to be. Stick to the basics, give them a good try, and remember to enjoy the ride. After all, you get to learn more about yourself.

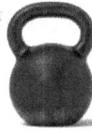

PART 2

Meaningful Goals Create Motivation

BREAKING FREE OF LOW MOTIVATION

Not every training session has to be an amazing feat worthy of a Facebook update. You don't need to invade the gym like it's Normandy and the weights are the Axis powers. Training like this leads to disappointment and burnout, both of which will hurt your efforts towards a positive and sustainable change.

You will achieve sustainable change when, day after day, you show up and do what you were meant to do that day. Most training sessions are average; some are plain awful; and a few are phenomenal, worthy of a self-high-five and an imitation of the moonwalk. But the sooner you accept that moonwalk-moments are rare, the more satisfied you'll be.

Your health and fitness life shouldn't be operated by an on/off switch, but rather by a dial that you tune depending on what is happening in your life at a given time. If you turn it off completely, you'll have to muster all your strength to start over again from zero momentum. You have to build all those habits again from a pile of shattered resolutions.

When you start a new training program, join a new gym or decide that this time you will lose five kilograms, it will be exciting in the beginning. Nothing can stop you! The mistake that most of us make is that we think this motivation will last forever. In reality, it will last about six weeks, if you're lucky. That's when things get hard. You'll get a life-style-change hangover. Be ready for it. Know that this amazing feeling won't last. The resolution that was exciting and new becomes an old thing. A bland, boring, same-old-same-old, routine. And what's more boring than a routine?

Nothing.

No matter how special and driven you are, you too will exhaust your limited resources of motivation. But it's OK; it happens to everyone once the excitement of the new wears off.

Getting over the hangover

Acknowledge that training and new habits will make you feel uncomfortable. Learn why discomfort will happen, and know that it is normal. Knowing this will reduce your stress, anxiety and fear. And when you expect discomfort, it will affect you less. It won't hit you like a 10-ton hammer every single time. And by keeping the routine alive during the shit times, you keep a small fire burning until you are ready to pour the gasoline on again. It's easier to get things blazing from a small fire than it is to start a new one.

I've been training since I was a 15-year-old snot face, battling vocal chord changes with way too much gel in my hair. (Hey, spikes were a thing, once.) Still, to this day I go through unmotivated periods in training. And yes, it's as much fun as rubbing sawdust into your eyes. But I've got a secret tool to re-motivate myself.

Motivation = Discipline = Motivation

When motivation and the initial excitement fades, I remind myself: *motivation is discipline.* This is something I got from listening to retired Navy SEAL Jocko Willink in his *Jocko Podcast.* Accepting this can feel like discovering the truth about Santa Claus. But it is also liberating. It means that you are responsible for your own actions, and therefore motivation. No longer can you wake up in the morning and not do a task because you are not motivated to do so. You have to admit that you don't have the discipline to do it this morning.

If you let motivation (and its daily fluctuations) drive your behaviour, you'll forever be at its mercy. Your actions will follow what you *feel* like doing instead of what you have to get done. You need discipline to build consistency and get results over time. You don't get that by waiting for the next wave of motivation to rise.

Training won't always be fun, exciting or something to look forward to with the drive of a rooster released in a barnyard of chickens. Too often we expect everything in life to be fun. Yet, work can be a grind; saving money feels like deprivation from all the awesome things you could buy now. In the same way, training can be batshit boring and weekly meal prep as much fun as giving birth to a two dozen golf balls through your nostril. But none of the fruit-bearing actions of life need to be fun every single day of the year. You don't skip work just because you don't feel like it today, or because the project you're working on isn't fun. You keep showing up to your office because you need to pay the mortgage and feed the kids. You save money because you know you need to have a safety net for rainy days. I know, I'd rather spend it on champagne and a cruise in the Mediterranean too.

Let's use the same thinking when training and healthy eating are not exciting. You do them because you know you need to. It's like putting money in the Bank of Health for the future. You build your health the same way you build your career. It's part of living a healthy life, whether it's fun or not. And before you know it, a new wave of excitement, motivation and enthusiasm will appear on the horizon. Keep the momentum going with discipline until then.

Motivation increases as we make and keep promises to ourselves. The size of the promise doesn't matter. By doing what you said you'd do, you'll empower yourself for future success. You'll increase your awareness of self-control and license yourself to accept more responsibility for your life. When you hold on to your promises, you build integrity and become a person who does what they said they'd do. As much as you want motivation to be something that you'll get from somewhere else, it has to come from within you.

I often see folks struggle with discipline because they're focusing on goals and activities that don't align with their deeper values. The analogy that the productivity wizard Stephen R Covey uses in *The 7 Habits of Highly Effective People* is that you'll end up climbing the wrong ladder. It's challenging to climb a ladder that doesn't lead to something that truly matters to you. If you've been struggling with discipline lately, you may need to reassess your goals. Once you have a goal that you truly want to achieve, you will have not only the motivation, but also the discipline to do it. And that's not the quick fix answer that most people want to hear.

WHAT ARE YOU WILLING TO GIVE UP?

There's a problem a lot of people ignore when goal setting, and that's the hardship that the road to the goal will lash upon them. What do we have to give up in order to reach our goal? How much hardship lies between point A and point B? And most importantly, are we willing endure it?

We admire the flashy end result of someone else's journey and often forget or choose to ignore the sacrifices they've made. We forget that achieving a certain goal requires us to step outside what we consider comfortable. If you want to lose 20 kg but are not willing to sacrifice your nightly ice-cream habit, we have a problem. If you want to cut down on drinking but don't want to stop going to the pub with your mates after a day's work, we have a problem. If you want to shred like Father Slash but can't endure the initial finger hurt, we have a problem. You get the idea.

I bet you know people who are drastically overweight and struggling with their health, yet they know everything there is to know about healthy eating. They are walking encyclopaedias of diet information, but they frequent the place with golden arches where fries are served by clowns. They are knowledge hoarders with no true intention of using the information wisely. Now, I understand that sometimes there are issues beyond just willingness. But unfortunately it still holds true for some.

This is because goal setting is the easy part. All you have to do is put words on paper. The hard part is coming to terms with the fact that something has to give, and you will have to suffer for your goals. Are you willing to go through that? If not, look for another goal or you'll end up going in circles. Why do you think so many people set health goals and never get anywhere? They are not willing to sacrifice. They are too comfortable where they are, with no desire to leave the Shire because it might mean walking through Mordor.

My advice? Don't try to make things perfect. A lot of people struggle as they try to make grand changes that won't last. Even if something feels like a worthless change, it's not. It's a start. It's better to lose one kilogram a year than not to lose anything at all. It's better to save $100 a year than to have no savings at all.

There's no right or wrong here. But stop kidding yourself about what you are willing to work for.

Write down three things you are willing to give up for your health and fitness goals:

1.

2.

3.

REASONS FOR LOW MOTIVATION

How many times in the past have you gotten excited about starting a new exercise routine, diet plan, daily meditation or some other mind-bending and body-transforming activity? And how many times have you stopped before things properly took off? If times of low motivation are frequent in your life, it might be worth digging deeper and discovering why your motivation keeps fading. As motivation for each person is different and the list of reasons it may fade are as wide as the sky, the following is by no means comprehensive. But these are the most common issues I've come across with clients (and myself, for that matter).

1. You want it but don't need it

Before you fall into deep self-pity, thinking you've failed at life for giving up on a healthy habit, know that this is completely normal. We've all set out to do something in the past only to stop when things get tough, complicated or when we just simply get bored of doing it. Yet none of this is fixed by acquiring more willpower so you can soldier on: it's about taking a deeper look at what you are doing.

This used to happen to me all the time when starting a new training program that didn't go hand in hand, on a deeper level, with what I wanted from my training. The training plan looked great on paper, but after a week or two I'd be sick of it. Not physically sick, but "meh" sick. Bored.

It was because I wanted something from the cycle of training but I didn't really *need* it. Yet I went years without understanding it. I kept jumping from program to program and going on and off eating plans. I was like a crow chasing a silver spoon. I really wanted the spoon but, to be honest, I didn't need it for anything. It served no purpose except something superficial. When I let go of the thought of wanting the spoon, took a step back and decided what I *needed* from training, things changed. I understood that the spoon had no value for me, and I stopped wanting it.

If you have been struggling with your health your whole life, starting and stopping more times than you care to count, you probably want to get healthier. But if you are not making progress, it may not be something that you really *need* at this point. Sure, it would be nice to be leaner, stronger and have better blood sugar levels, but it's not necessary for you today.

Things usually change for people when they get a serious diagnosis of some sort. Most people do a 180 degree U-turn once they receive the ultimatum of "do this, or else". That's when the want becomes a *need*. Yet, it's always better to work on prevention than waiting for your health to take a deep downturn before commencing damage control.

2. You are relying on outside sources for motivation

Now, I'm sure I had to work hard to pull you out of your social media feed to read this book. Even with promises of help for your lack of motivation, most of us would just rather scroll the feed for pretty pictures with motivational quotes. Maybe you think arming yourself with inspirational quotes and pictures of oiled specimens is what gives you the kick in the ass that you need.

No personal trainer or fitness feed in social media can keep you motivated by pushing you into a certain direction. Sure, another person can help you to find and unleash the motivation within you. But it is not something that is done *to* you. Rather, it is something that involves painful levels of soul-searching, with or without help from another person. And it takes a lot more than internet memes. I get it;

it's effortless to scroll the photos. But here's something you probably know but don't want to admit: they don't work. Entertaining to read, yes. Effective for long-term motivation, nope. As a matter of fact, the photos might do the opposite by reducing your motivation. They could make you feel like you're too far from where you want to be, which leads us to reason 3 below.

3. You are trying to do something that is too far beyond your level of competence

If you've never done any training and jump straight into lifting four days a week, expect it to be hard. Now, if you didn't show up on the third day, you will feel as if you've failed because you are not doing what you set out to do. Even though, despite missing one training session, you're still doing way more than you did a week ago. Unfortunately we tend to see what we are *not* doing rather than what we *are* doing.

A better way to go about the change is to start just beyond your current level of competence. Instead of planning to train four days per week, start with two training sessions. You have to feel like you are winning. Things get unmotivated real fast if you move from one failure to another, even if you are actually doing better than before.

When deciding on a new habit, I encourage you to pick something which you are at least 90% sure you can succeed at. I got that tip from the great people and motivation experts of Habitry. Anything less than 90% and you are choosing a new habit that is too hard, unless the stars perfectly align (which they never do). Your life, most likely, has other things going on as well: you have a job, maybe you are a parent, and you might even own a pet parrot that needs your attention. Can you succeed with your habit on days when your pet parrot is rattling its cage by doing somersaults and screaming profanities to get your attention? I know I couldn't. And I don't even know any parrots.

4. You are being dictated to

In order to stay motivated, you need to feel personally responsible for your actions and behaviours. And these behaviours need to be aligned with your values. There's a fancy words for this: *autonomy*.

When a new client comes to me for advice, I don't dictate strict rules that they must follow. That might work in the short term, but it rarely brings a long-lasting solution into their lifestyle. It doesn't have any autonomy built into it. That's why, when I first meet a new client, I like to ask what they value in life. This gives me an idea about what drives their desire for change. If you have a track record of stopping change before it even properly starts, you need to dig into your values before starting yet another fitness plan. More on that later.

5. You are yet to discover why you want to accomplish what you set out to do

You need to know why you are doing what you are doing. Your *why* is the main engine for your motivation. Start by asking yourself why you want to make these changes. In what ways would your life be better if you made these changes?

Even with the above sorted, there will be times when motivation is not quite as ripe and ready for picking as it could be. During those times it's good to build routines and habits into your daily life that can carry you through.

ALIGN YOUR GOALS WITH YOUR VALUES

Train to be better at life. Don't train for the sake of being better at training. That's a twist on the Dan John quote, "Fitness is the ability to do a task". Nothing else.

Fitness shouldn't be something that restricts your life – quite the opposite. Fitness should give you increased energy, stamina and strength to chase and accomplish whatever it is that is important to you. And if you start looking better in the process, that's a bonus.

Base your training and life goals on the values that you hold close to your heart. It's important to discover or revisit your values now instead of just putting meaningless goals on a piece of paper. When you base your goals on what society, your family, friends, co-workers or SpongeBob consider to be "good", but ignore what you really believe in, you will be pushing water uphill for the rest of your life. You will feel like you are failing at everything because you are trying to get somewhere you really don't care about going.

How to get the most out of this exercise

1. Depending on the time of the day, pour yourself something along the lines of:

- a big cup of coffee. I like mine strong and black, ideally with notes of chocolate.

- good quality single-malt Scotch. Anything from the fine folk at Highland Park is worth exploring.

- sparkling water with fresh lime. You know, when you've had too much coffee and Scotch.

2. Find a place where you won't be bothered for the next 90 minutes.

3. Get a pen and answer the questions below. I prefer a pen instead of typing, as the answers burn deeper into your brain with handwriting. There's research on this, somewhere. Trust me.

4. File the answers away and come back to them in a few days' time to see if you'd like to add or change anything. These answers are not locked in for the rest of your life. They might change as you evolve, so keep on exploring.

Question 1: What do you value in life?

When your training and health goals don't match your values you will continuously find yourself stopping and starting exercise routines. Case in point, I spent my late teens and the majority of my twenties trying to put on as much muscle as I possibly could. I failed, over and over again. And I restarted as many times. I pursued this goal, occasionally achieving results but more often failing for 15 years because I used to believe that to be a man I had to look a certain way. I was trying to fit into a mould that the fitness culture had created.

One day, I wrote down what I valued: health and longevity, strength, quality time with friends and family, cooking with my then-girlfriend (now wife), good food, music, history, travel …

It took me close to 15 years to realise that I kept struggling and failing because getting yoked wasn't what I valued in life. Fifteen years of frustration – chasing and failing at a goal I didn't actually value! Sure, I still want to look good. But I don't obsess over it enough to count calories or say no to having a good time. Hopefully that convinced you enough to write down your values – saving you 15 years of frustration in the process.

Write your values here:

Question 2: Why are you doing this?

What is the driver behind your desire for a healthier lifestyle? What are you looking to get out of it? What's the end goal and how is this going to make your life better once you are successfully practising healthier habits?

If you struggle for ideas here are some common answers I hear:

- I want my partner to find me attractive again.
- I want to have more and/or better sex, have more stamina and energy.
- I want to be a better role model for my kids.
- I want to reduce my anxiety, improve mental health and happiness.*
- I want to look after my family and be someone they can rely on.
- I want to have more energy so can I do more of the things that make me happy.
- I want to improve my confidence so I can live a fuller life.
- I want to improve longevity – to be able to do tomorrow what I can do today.

*Please, please, please seek professional help if you struggle with anxiety or other mental health issues.

There is no one right answer here. No matter what your reason for training is, it will be the right one for you. Use this to your advantage. Write your reasons below and don't move forward until you've drilled this down. Seeking the answers should make you a little uncomfortable.

Write why you are doing this:

Question 3: Who are you doing this for?

Are you doing this for yourself or for someone else? Is it because it will improve your life or the lives of those around you – your partner, kids or perhaps friends? It helps to think of how you or others will be affected if you keep ignoring your health.

Write who you are doing this for:

"But I don't know what I want"

You don't always have to know what you want. Sometimes it can be helpful to ask yourself what you don't want. Take the opposite approach instead of trying to search for the ultimate answer. Take me for example. Occasionally I don't know what I want to focus on with my training. I can't come up with a single big goal to train for. Nothing really inspires me enough to dive headfirst into a challenge or a training program. But when I flip the question to "What is it that I don't want?", the previously murky water now has a bit of clarity.

I don't want to train, look or eat purely for aesthetics. I don't want to be sore and injured. I don't want to count calories or worry about having a few beers on the weekend. I don't want to do weights for more than four days a week or more than 60 minutes at a time.

Just by making a list of "don't wants" I've eliminated quite a few things. Even if I don't know exactly what I want to train for, I've given myself a bit of direction.

Sometimes it's OK to not have specific goals.

Write down what you absolutely <u>do not want:</u>

WHEN YOUR GOALS BECOME OVERWHELMING

Setting yourself a big goal might not be the most effective technique for some people. I've found that having grand goals can sometimes deter people from taking any action at all. In those cases, focusing on "process goals" is a great way to achieve larger goals that might at first seem too intimidating. A process goal gives you a clear pathway to follow. You either achieve the process goal, or you don't. There's no *maybes, buts* or *one days*. You just follow what you set out to do.

Establishing your guiding values will help you set process goals here, just as it did in the previous exercise. You'll find my values-driven process goals below.

Once you accept that goals and interests change over time, and just let your values guide you, it's easier to let go of the grand, overwhelming goals. Instead, all you have to focus on is the question: Did I achieve my process goal for today?

I value: Physical health – to move well, be pain-free and avoid typical lifestyle diseases

Process goals:

- Spend 5 minutes taking my joints through the full ranges of motion daily. The older we get, the quicker we lose mobility in any body part not being regularly used.

- Strength train 2–4 times per week.

- Do a longer walk or other activity 1–3 times a week.

⊙ Keep my body composition in check by eating mostly wholefoods at least 90% of the time.

I value: Psychological health – to be the best version of myself I can be and to reduce mental deterioration once old(er)

Process goals:

⊙ Meditate every morning for 10 minutes.

⊙ Learn at least one new thing each day, no matter how insignificant it seems.

⊙ Listen to music each day.

⊙ Play guitar for at least 10 minutes a day, 3–4 days a week. (I've made picking up my guitar a very low-barrier goal. Most days that I play, I practise for much longer than 10 minutes. But if I made the goal *play for an hour each day,* I'd never pick it up.)

⊙ Stop and practise mindfulness and gratitude at least once in the morning and once before going to bed.

I value: Meaningful relationships – because good people make me feel good

Process goals:

⊙ Analyse opportunities and commitments based on how they could affect my relationship with my wife. If they are likely to have a negative effect on our relationship with no long-term benefit, they are not worth pursuing.

- Be actively present during conversations – with everyone. (This is hard!)

- Don't associate with dickheads.

I value: Freedom

Process goals:

- Choose freedom over money – this guides most of my decisions. For example, I'd make more money by training clients on Mondays and Saturdays but I prefer to have the freedom to pursue other things on those days.

- Say *no* to things that I don't value, even if it means missing out.

I value: Meaningful work – to make the world a better place

Process goals:

- Before each session with a client I ask myself: What one thing can I do to help this person today?

- Don't bitch and moan about my day to my clients. When a client sees me, I want that time to be one of the highlights of their day, not something that they dread.

- Use my blog to share what I've learned and what has worked for my clients so my readers can improve themselves.

All of the actions that go with the values above have a fair amount of flexibility in them. And this is the hardest part to grasp: all of the values don't have to be in balance every day. As long as the values stay more or less in balance over a course of a week, month or year, it's all good.

Note: It took me a long time to build up my process goals and habits to this point. I didn't start by focusing on all of these at once. And I don't nail all of these process goals all the time; sometimes I struggle with them too. However, there are definitely some non-negotiable things on this list that I get done, no matter what.

Steps for creating process goals

1. Write down five areas in your life that are important to you: things that you hold valuable. I am not talking about writing down single majestic words like "purity, elegance, holiness". Rather, write *what* is important to you.

2. Follow each answer from the first question with *why* this is important to you.

3. Write down one practical action that will honour each important thing. This becomes your process goal.

I would suggest that focusing on only one process goal at a time is the way to go. When you try to dig too many holes at once, none of them are deep enough, making you feel unaccomplished and running the risk of becoming discouraged. It takes patience, but that's the secret to success with most things.

Write down five things that you value in your life, followed by <u>one</u> practical action that becomes your process goal. Nail one process goal at a time.

1.

2.

3.

4.

5.

ACCEPT OWNERSHIP OF YOUR HEALTH

To maximise long-term success with your health and fitness it is crucial to take ownership of your situation. Think of yourself as a student of health and fitness. Even when you are busy and occupied with other things in life, don't just show up and mindlessly do what you are told, then forget all about it until your next session. Rather, pay attention at each training session and have the mindset that you will teach a friend some of the things that you have learned, or observe as if you have to take a test to answer questions regarding your training and nutrition.

Sure, this is harder than just showing up, but it will serve you in many ways. You will have control and knowledge of your situation instead of blindly believing what's put in front of you. Your "shit radar" will improve. This shit radar needs to be on full blast when sailing through all things health and fitness – an industry that is notoriously polluted with confusing information.

It is easier to learn a new habit or a skill when you teach it to someone else. Not only because you have to repeat what you've done but also because you are more likely to have success when working in teams or as a part of a larger community of people who have similar goals.

The emphasis should be on learning the principles and skills behind the method. It's not just a workout or a meal plan. It's an ongoing process of learning, provided that you keep an open mind. When you only learn a skill or a new exercise, you can only take it so far before eventually needing to progress. You know how to do something, but you have no idea why. Eventually you run out of choices. But when you learn the principle behind the concept and truly understand it, that's when you are in control of your situation.

The first option for you is to show up, blindly follow instructions, go home and forget everything. Repeat the same thing over and over again and never really learn anything on a deeper level. Or you can think of your health and fitness as a lifelong learning project. It's your body and your mind. Remember that no instructor, personal trainer, coach or anyone else knows your mind and your body like you do.

So which one are you, a lifelong student of your health and fitness or a sheep who blindly follows and believes everything that's put in front of them?

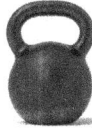

PART 3

There's Never Enough Time

STOP KILLING YOURSELF

Most of us are privileged enough to have been given a fully functioning and amazing piece of machinery at birth called the human body. Yet we complain about the hardship of exercise and movement like it's a burden, something that we *have to do.* We should be grateful that we are able to move and do all the great things in life that involve using our body to its full capacity. Some people with disabilities never get the chance to explore these possibilities.

We spend most of our youth doing all things imaginable to test the limits of our bodies. It's sad then that, as we hit adulthood, we start to forget what we've learned about movement. Paraphrasing world-renowned strength coach Mike Boyle, we end up sitting eight hours a day at work, a few hours during the daily commute and another few hours while watching television at night. We are practically reverting to the foetal position: being hunched up while sitting.

I understand that we all have to work and, for some, work involves extended periods of sitting. It's one of the curses of the modern world. But there are ways around it. Some of my clients have standing desks, and they are conscious of how much sitting they do during the day. If a standing desk is not an option at your workplace, you can try to get off your chair often during the day. Set alarms to remind you. Hold meetings standing up, if possible. While moving for an hour in the evening is great, what's even better is to take mini-breaks during the day to break up the sitting. Your body will thank you for it. Get on top of things before you have to. In other words, do it before it becomes an issue, before you end up in pain. Use it or lose it.

Ignoring your health is like buying the most expensive car, taking it to the rally derby and getting the shit bashed out of it. Sure, it's good fun while it lasts, but I wouldn't want to be the one repairing it. Or paying for it. The difference with cars, of course, is that you can buy a new one. But you've only got one body and it's meant to last you a lifetime. I am hoping you will make your lifetime a long one rather than a short one.

Relearn and explore movement: squat, run, roll around. Depending on your level and the amount of time you've spent in the foetal position, you might not be able to tackle the toughest movements right out of the gates, and that's fine. As long as you gradually challenge your body, you are heading in the right direction. Just move. Make it a habit.

If you are getting sick all the time or just feeling tired day in and day out, your body is trying to tell you something. Sure, everyone gets sick now and then; that's life. But if taking sick leave for you is as common as eating potatoes for dinner is for me, it's worth stopping for a second to ask yourself if you are taking care of your body the way it deserves. The way *you* deserve! You cannot keep ignoring the patterns, blaming the weather, the kids, or the shape of the moon on that particular evening in 2009. Rather, take a look in the mirror and ask, "What am I doing?"

Draw the lines, connect the dots. You only have *one single body* for the rest of your life. Look after it and do whatever you can to make it last.

After all that, just remember that it doesn't have to be an all-or-nothing situation. Unless you let it get that way before taking action, that is. You can still have a drink, eat a piece of cake and do all the other things in life you enjoy. Just balance it out with some frequent movement, plenty of vegetables and find ways to rest and relax.

As much as I hate clichés, you can't ignore that an ounce of prevention is worth a pound of cure. And it all starts now.

"I DON'T HAVE TIME"

When it comes to training or healthy cooking, one of the most common obstacles is time. Specifically, the lack of it. Maybe you've got kids, hobbies and a busy social life with friends. Then there's work, and I guess your partner needs some dedicated time too. I get it; you feel like there's not enough time in the day to fit everything in. Something's gotta give and often the first thing to go is the fitness routine. You hope to pick it up again once the schedule eases up a bit.

Yet, I am sure that at times you have been extremely busy and something important came up that just had to get done. Maybe you got invited to a party that you couldn't say no to. Or something urgent came up at work that needed attention yesterday. In those situations, somehow magically the extra time appears from thin air. How is it then that you struggle to fit exercise or healthy cooking into your day? They would have a tremendous, positive impact on your health.

Every so often it's worthwhile to self-audit your daily time usage. You might come across major "time leaks" in your days due to poor time-management habits: things such as checking Facebook or watching the news for the 10th time the same day. Or coming home after work and sitting on the couch for long enough to grow roots. It's even possible that you spend nine hours at work each day but only half of it is productive. The other half is spent socialising, reading unimportant emails, and reacting to problems instead of being proactive about them. I am certainly guilty of these and I often do them without realising.

How to find more time

I recommend keeping a detailed time diary for at least three days, but preferably a week, in order to see some patterns emerging. Pay close attention to what happens in the morning before going to work and in the evening after clocking out. But also carefully observe how you spend time while at work. Are you working hard? Or hardly working?

Download the workbook from **RepsAndTheRest.com/SpandexNot-Compulsory** and start a time diary tomorrow morning. If you live in the digital world this is also easy to do on Google Keep or similar.

One piece of advice before you start: write down *everything*. Try not to judge any actions or tasks you find yourself doing. Write them all down to get a full picture of what is happening during your day. Observation, not judgement, is what you are after.

Time diary

DATE:	TASK / ACTION
Time:	
Time:	
Time:	
Time:	
Time:	
Time:	
Time:	
Time:	
Time:	
Time:	
Time:	
Time:	
Time:	
Time:	
Time:	

A day out of my time diary

DATE: WED 26.7.17	TASK / ACTION
Time: 4:50 am	Get up, dress, feed the cats, brush teeth.
Time: 5:00 am	Put coffee on, do *Morning Movement Routine* while waiting
Time: 5:10 am	Pack coffee and food for the day (pre-made on Monday / night before)
Time: 5:15 am	Meditate

Time: 5:30am	Start commute to work (reading a book)
Time: 7:00 am	Clients
Time: 9:15 am	Breakfast (and talking to colleagues, deciding on what to do before the next lot of clients)
Time: 10:15 am	Café – working on this book
Time: 11.15 am	Clients
Time: 12 pm	Protein shake, peanut butter and banana sandwich for quick lunch
Time: 12:15 pm	Clients
Time: 2:30 pm	Internet, Facebook, procrastinating before training session
Time: 3:00 pm	Training session, shower, meal
Time: 4:45 pm	Work admin
Time: 5:50 pm	Commute
Time: 6:30 pm	Improv class
Time: 9:30 pm	Commute (internet, social media, music)
Time: 11:00 pm	Arrive home, get ready for bed (if I know I am getting home late I organise everything the day before so I can get to bed without too much of a delay)
Time: 11.20 pm	Sleep

Reflect on what you wrote down

As with keeping a diet diary, the value is to *objectively* be able to look back on your day written on a piece of paper. Seeing stuff written down works wonders. Make observations on how much time you spent on different tasks. Remember to be honest and detailed. Now it's time to see how your time spent matches with what you value in life. Once that's done, let's see how you could improve your time-management skills to align better with your values.

To give you an idea, I've given my answers below each question.

1. What do I value the most in life?

Quality time with my wife, my health, hobbies, friends, music, helping others.

2. How much time do I spend on things that I value?

On this particular day, I completely ignored my number one priority and value in life: spending quality time with my wife. In my defence, this is the only day in a week that I barely see the woman because I have my improv class in the evening.

Apart from that I did pretty good.

Health: ate well because I pre-cooked all my meals, got training done. Hobbies and friends: did three hours of improv with newly found friends. Music: listened to some on the train. But didn't get in any guitar practice. Helping others: plenty of clients, worked on this book.

3. In what ways do I waste time?

Because of our living situation, I spend a ridiculous amount of time commuting. I need to be adamant to not waste time while sitting on the train but focus on getting work done, or learn something from books or podcasts, especially in the morning when I have more energy. In the evenings I listen to music and try to relax. I try not to waste time on the internet / social media.

5. What changes could I make so my days would reflect my values?

I could be more effective during breakfast / late afternoon meal and not linger around our staffroom as much. But sometimes this brings up interesting conversations with people too. So it's not all shit.

Get the training session done straight after the last client instead of procrastinating.

Not every day is like this. Some days I am more effective and some days I barely get anything done apart from seeing clients. I only commute four days a week so on other days I have more non-travel time to spare too.

Not everything that you value has to be accomplished every single day. Some days you'll pay attention to some aspects of life and other days to others. As long as you keep a balance when looking at the big picture of a week, month, or even a year, you can be happy with that. That's what having a balanced life is all about.

Start implementing small changes

Start by changing 15 minutes a day. Maybe it's as easy as getting up as soon as the alarm goes off instead of snoozing. Or having three coffees with colleagues instead of four. Once the first change becomes somewhat "automated", you are ready for another minor change.

I know you have a lot of things going on in your life. You're busy. But we all have the same 24 hours and that is not going to change anytime soon. Make the most out of what you've got and match the time spent with your values and life goals. There's nothing worse than wasting time. You're never going get any of it back.

THE QUADRANTS OF TIME MANAGEMENT

If there is one thing I hear more than anything else it's, "Joonas, what kind of conditioner do you use for your hair?" But that's not what this chapter is about. My second-most-often-heard sentence is, "Joonas, I am too busy to exercise". Finding and committing time to training can be challenging, especially if your enjoyment level of exercise is somewhere on par with getting a root canal done at the dentist. However, I am yet to meet anyone who doesn't enjoy the feeling after the fact, or can flat-out deny that moving regularly hasn't made a difference to their body and mind.

Let's be honest here. It's rare that you don't have any time for exercise. Rather, you value other things more than movement so you are reacting to arising issues and pushing the scheduled training to the bottom of the list. I am not asking you to throw everything out and make training your number one priority. But if you can get exercise to be your fourth or fifth priority, after family, friends and work, well, now we're getting somewhere.

So how do we prioritise better? Effectiveness guru Stephen R Covey, the author of *The 7 Habits of Highly Effective People*, talked about four quadrants of time management. I've taken the liberty of making this more relevant for us.

Q1: Important and Urgent

These are the tasks that need to be done now. Or yesterday. The crises that we react to as they arise and that make us feel good to complete. But reacting to things is a poor way of managing time, and far from effective.

It's easy to fall into doing tasks at Q1 because it feels like you are doing the busy work and ticking things off the list. But you are often reacting to matters that are important to other people, not necessarily to you or to your long-term plan. You might think you are the captain of the ship; but truthfully, you are someone else's shitkicker.

Answering emails and ticking things off to-do lists often fall into this quadrant.

Q2: Important and Non-Urgent

This quadrant includes complicated tasks that have a positive impact for the future (when done right): think of training, exercise, cooking healthy meals and tracking health markers. These tasks involve planning and prevention. Because the results are not usually immediate, a lot of people put off tasks that reside in this quadrant.

Q3: Non-Important and Urgent

This quadrant houses distractions and interruptions that are not important but which still grab your attention. Think of the little red notification flags that come up on your phone or social media which trigger an "urgent" response and stop you from doing whatever important work you were previously doing. The Kardashian generation seem to be making their mark in this quadrant.

Q4: Non-Important and Non-Urgent

This quadrant holds time-wasting activities, like scrolling and obsessing over other person's Facebook feed or watching *The Kardashians.*

Q3 and Q4 categories are easy to fall into because most of the tasks are somewhat pleasant or enjoyable.

Ignoring health will increase the time spend in Q1 activities

It all comes down to what Covey calls your *product (P) / product capacity (PC) balance.* With health it means your body is the *P* and what you can do with your body is *PC*. If all you do is focus on the *PC* while ignoring your *P* you will eventually run into a dead end. You will milk your body (beautiful image, you're welcome) for all its resources while failing to maintain it as well as you can. Over time, this means less productivity, not only at work, but also less enjoyment of other aspects of your life outside of work.

If you keep ignoring your health and daily movement practices, Q1 activities will start to come up more often. You will get sick (and need to react to this illness), you will move poorly, feel tight and sore, and might even be in pain (you'll need to react to this by resting or by getting physical therapy), you will feel like crap since you are not sleeping enough (you'll need to make a speedball to stay awake). Ignoring Q2 is like fixing the leaking roof problem with a bucket instead of actually sealing the ceiling with a silicon sealant (say that fast 10 times).

ADJUSTING TRAINING AND EATING HABITS FOR LIFELONG SUCCESS

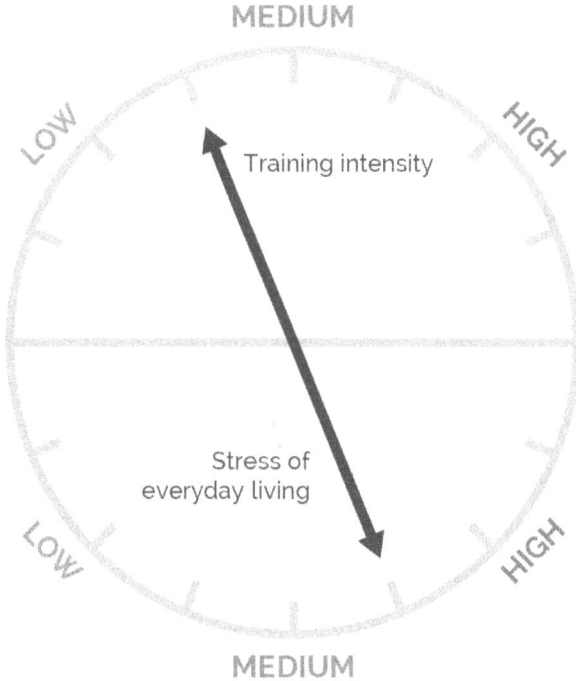

Your approach to health and fitness should not be operated by an on/ off button, but by a dial. On a dial, you can choose your level of intensity at any given time. At times you'll want to crank it up. And at other times you'll have to dial it down to the absolute minimum to deal with other things in life. Quiet at work and extra time to rest and recover? Turn the fitness dial up. Big project at work, sick child or overseas holiday? Turn the dial down and get only the minimum done. But for the most part, your aim is to keep your dial somewhere in the middle.

It doesn't sound exciting. And it sure doesn't sound like what the majority of the fitness industry and Instagram celebrities want you to believe. The fitness industry doesn't sell moderation. The industry thrives on selling you quick results, trying to make you believe that "going hardcore" is how you get anywhere. It's trying to guilt you into buying our products while selling training as a punishment for a life lived in the sin of gluttony and slothfulness. But using the dial works. Adjusting your training intensity to fit your life leads to sustainable, lifelong health. You might even get a six-pack. Just kidding. But I am part of the fitness industry so had to convince you somehow. Six-packs are over-rated.

Know when to pull back

These are the times when you're already chasing your tail, trying to catch life's curveballs as they are hit your way. There are work or family responsibilities that take priority, and you lack time or energy for health and fitness.

WHAT TO DO WITH TRAINING DURING PULL-BACK TIMES

Do the minimum to maintain what you've got so far. If you are used to training five hours a week, take it back to two or three, or even fewer. During pull-back times you are recovering and taking time off, because your body needs it. Stay active in other ways. You could go for a long walk, or work on flexibility and joint mobility for 20 minutes. Set aside a few minutes each day for mindfulness or another form of stress release.

WHAT *NOT* TO DO WITH TRAINING DURING PULL-BACK TIMES

Don't stress if you can't keep up with your normal training schedule. Don't tackle the new(est) *Hollywood Belly Fat Blaster* or *Gunz of He-Man* (by the people who brought you *Guns of Navarone*) training plans.

WHAT TO DO WITH DIET AND HABITS DURING PULL-BACK TIMES

Organise pre-cooked meals that can be heated with no effort. If your pull-back situation took you by surprise, you need to keep your cooking simple, efficient and nutritious. But tasty, too, so you'll actually eat what you're cooking. Cook big batches or find restaurants or delivery services that can cater to your diet needs.

Make it as simple as possible to maintain the habits you've worked for so far. As always, if you have the option to do so, planning trumps everything else.

WHAT *NOT* TO DO WITH DIET AND HABITS DURING PULL-BACK TIMES

Too many people resort to fast food and microwave dinners during these hectic periods. It's unfortunate, since you might already be stressed or tired and pushing your mental and physical limits. Piling poor dietary choices on top will make you feel lethargic, and you won't be at your best when others might need your superhuman skills. Don't worry about winning any Michelin stars with your cooking. Or mastering advanced vegetable chopping skills. Good enough is enough.

Don't add new habits unless you are 100% confident you can stick with them.

Know when to aim for reasonable progress

This is where we find ourselves most of the time. You might be busy balancing family, work, training and hobbies. You work normal hours on most days, and there's room for regular training in your schedule. Things are not chaotic or out of control. If chaos is your constant companion I suggest re-reading the previous chapters about time management.

WHAT TO DO WITH TRAINING DURING REASONABLE PROGRESS

It's good to alternate between easy and moderate training while occasionally, when the stars align, testing your limits. Stay *reasonable*. Show up and get your training done, then move on. Don't bang the dumbbells together trying to ignite the fire or get into a fistfight because someone else is using the 24 kg kettlebell. Try to progress during these times by doing a bit better each session.

Have flexibility built into your training so that you can adjust it if a situation arises at work or at home. Some weeks you might train more and on other weeks you might train less. As long as it all balances out over a longer period, it's all good. Think of your training as a lifelong marathon, not a six-week sprint.

WHAT *NOT* TO DO WITH TRAINING DURING REASONABLE PROGRESS

Don't be a hero and try to tackle epic and complicated training plans that are going to get thrown out the window as soon as something unexpected happens. Don't sign up for a "16 weeks to a 10-pack" boot camp.

You don't have to feel as if you've been run over by a freight train after each session.

WHAT TO DO WITH DIET AND HABITS DURING REASONABLE PROGRESS

Add and track new habits one at a time until they become part of your routine. Keep working on the habits that you have formed in the past and figure out ways to make them better suited for you. Plan ahead and know how to react when an unusual or stressful situation comes around.

WHAT *NOT* TO DO WITH DIET AND HABITS DURING REASONABLE PROGRESS

Don't take on habits unless you are at least 80–90% confident that you can succeed with them.

Know when to attack it like a bat out of hell

These are the times when work life is easy or non-existent. You have a private chef (or a very supportive partner, or mum) cooking all your meals and helping you with every request. You have a nanny with a British accent who looks after the kids while you overhead press in the penthouse. You might even own a pool. Possibly a dolphin too. Or you might be an 18-year-old living in your parents' basement. You have no money issues, work troubles or dependants to look after. What you do have is all the time in the world. Also, your dad is Gene Simmons.

WHAT TO DO WITH TRAINING DURING THESE TIMES

Always wanted to try the hardest of all training plans? Want to tackle the insane six-month plan that The Rock is on? Spend an extra hour at the gym each day just to work on your triceps? Go for it, this is your chance.

WHAT *NOT* TO DO WITH TRAINING DURING THESE TIMES

Don't try to break the world record for squatting on a stability ball, because, well, it's just dumb. And dangerous. Otherwise, do whatever you want. Because, why not? Nothing is going to slow you down.

WHAT TO DO WITH DIET AND HABITS DURING THESE TIMES

Go on the strictest eating plan and calculate and weigh every single calorie and macronutrient. Let your life revolve around eating, and skip every possible social gathering in order to become the version of yourself that you want to be. I mean, for you, success is measured in weights lifted and protein consumed.

WHAT *NOT* TO DO WITH DIET AND HABITS DURING THESE TIMES

Don't search for the secret supplement to increase your arm size. Don't eat magic mushrooms or go on a juice cleanse to lose weight. Also, don't do steroids or take diet pills.

By now, you might have realised that for most of us the last scenario is as rare as feeding hay to a double-headed donkey. It is unlikely that you will be so fortunate. (Then again, maybe you are a bored 18-year-old billionaire living in your parents' basement with your dolphin, high-fiving Gene Simmons.)

The times that are ideal for combining a tough training plan with a strict diet might come along once a year, at best. Yet, this is what most people do when they start a journey toward their fitness goals. They sign up for mad challenges or follow a training and diet plan they found online. Those plans are designed for someone who has the luxury to train for a living, or for those who have some form of chemical adjustments flowing through their veins. This is why most normal people who start them, fail.

You are going to have more success by adhering to a reasonable and well-balanced approach that can be adjusted to fit your life as it changes. Sometimes you'll do more and sometimes you'll do less. Occasionally, you'll just work on staying where you are without worrying about progress. Hell, at times you might even regress a bit. I mean, I enjoy training more than most people, but it's not my whole life. It's just one part of it. Reasonable progress doesn't sound sexy or sell a lot of books or make great TV programs, but it does work better, if you have the patience for it. And if you do it consistently over a long period of time, the results will stick.

ODD ROUTINES TO IMPROVE TIME MANAGEMENT AND HEALTH

Oh, routines. Tell me more about how boring your life is. But wait! It doesn't have to be so. When people complain that they don't have time to exercise or eat healthy it's often (and again) a sign of poor time management. And (a good) routine is the king of time management. Maybe some people can wing life but I'm lost when I don't have my routines in place. I find that without routines I'm just reacting to the stuff that happens around me, instead of proactively seizing the day.

Routines are a base for a healthy body

Building life around positive routines allows us to focus on what's important and worth doing. We could waste countless hours each week on unimportant decisions like what to wear, what to have for breakfast or what to do in the gym. This time is lost from activities that truly matter, like spending quality time with loved ones, exercising with a purpose, making healthier decisions about food, or just generally having a good time.

I believe that if we are relying on small and meaningless decisions to bring excitement to our lives, we are not getting the big picture. Streamlining these small decisions creates space and time for what's important. Here are some ways that I've streamlined my life over the past few years.

MINIMALIST WARDROBE

I used to be terrible at deciding what to wear. Now it takes me 5 minutes, flat. And that's on a bad day. To streamline, I decided to only wear black 98% of the time. The other 2% is mostly dark blue and grey. What can I say; I'm practically a rainbow. I never have an issue involving a certain shirt not going with a pair of pants. Everything in my wardrobe goes with everything. Instead of a hundred different combinations of clothing that never gets worn, my minimalist wardrobe is easy and practical. Also, wearing mostly black is a lot less confusing for someone who's colourblind.

TWICE-A-YEAR WARDROBE CLEAN-UP

Every six months I go through my wardrobe and pile up any items that I haven't worn at least five times. Then I take that pile of clothing to charity. It's liberating to eliminate clutter. I also went through 2016 without buying any new clothing, which helped me to see which items I wear most. At the end of the year the maths was simple: buy more of the things I wear and get rid of the rest.

GETTING UP AT 4:50 AM SIX DAYS A WEEK

I don't set the alarm for Sundays but I am usually up before 7 am anyway ... unless I've had one too many single malts the night before. This routine allows me to read and write each morning before Colleen gets up. I write and think better when it's dark and quiet and everyone else is still asleep. Some people can work and write in cafes but I need peace and quiet.

ONLY BLACK COFFEE FOR THE FIRST 4–5 HOURS
AFTER WAKING UP

"OMG, Joonas, don't you know that breakfast is the most important meal of the day and that every time you skip breakfast a puppy will be shot into space?" Yes, I hear that a lot. But I've found that for me, not eating during the first part of the day has taught me to dissociate between real hunger and the mental feeling of "I need to eat". I am better at making food choices even when hungry because I can make rational decisions instead of eating whatever is in sight. In the West, we live in a world where food is available to us 24/7, so we've forgotten how it feels to experience hunger. It's good to remind ourselves every once in a while that it's OK not to eat. I am not going to die if I don't eat every three hours. It's about conditioning the body and mind.

Not eating also allows me to focus on reading or writing in the morning instead of worrying about what to eat. I feel like I think more clearly with just black coffee in my system first thing in the morning. And by the way, this has nothing to do with calorie control since I eat plenty during the rest of the day. If you are used to eating every two to three hours, you could start by adding slightly longer periods between meal times. It might even make you healthier. There's plenty of fasting research to back it up.

Word of caution: fasting doesn't necessarily work for everyone. Some women especially seem to react poorly to prolonged fasting. And if you have any medical conditions or history with eating disorders, discuss your health goals with a doctor.

BED BY 9.45 PM EVERY NIGHT

I follow this religiously unless I've been out seeing a gig or something else special, because I know my body requires a good sleep to give me enough energy for the next day. In order to get to sleep easily I try not to use any electronics for an hour or so before bed, and I read a physical book (as in, made out of paper) not requiring too much brain power which helps me to switch off. Full disclosure: I am extremely gifted at falling asleep at night.

COOKING AND FOOD PREP ON MONDAYS

Depending on the week ahead, this might take one hour or closer to three. No, I don't always enjoy cooking and, yes, it's time away from other, more enjoyable, tasks. But it pays dividends throughout the week. I know what I have for lunches and dinners and I don't have to spend an hour cooking after a long day of work. Besides, the better I eat, the better I feel, so this is worth my time every week. I go a step further here and usually have a few different dishes for lunches that I rotate from week to week. I don't mind eating the same meals for lunch when it's convenient and healthy. Dinners can then be more exciting or at least something different.

If you know how to cook some healthy, quick and easy meals and they taste decent, why not stick to them instead of trying to reinvent the wheel each week? You can even cook massive batches that'll last you two weeks. This way you'll only need to cook every fortnight.

If I fail to cook before the start of the week, I'll be chasing my tail until Saturday.

Side note: "Leftovers" is my favourite meal because it means I don't have to cook. Buy a dozen or so pyrex containers (the IKEA brand is cheaper but they chip easily). Each time you cook a meal, quadruple the recipe and save the leftovers. Just keep the veggies on the side and cook them fresh each time you reheat a container of food, unless you're into soggy vegetables.

ONLY CHECK EMAIL TWICE A DAY

I used to open my email about 20 times a day to check if there was something there. Now, I am no mathematician but this shit adds up over time. I was wasting time reacting to non-urgent incoming messages when there were more important tasks I had to get done. It would constantly stop my workflow. Now I check my email mid-morning or noon and once in the evening, unless I am waiting for something urgent to come through. This was a game changer. And yes, sometimes I still fail at it.

LIMIT FACEBOOK (AND ANY OTHER SOCIAL MEDIA) USE

I've turned off all the notifications and alerts. I've installed News Feed Eradicator for Facebook on Chrome that blocks my news feed. I've uninstalled the Facebook app on my phone and tablet. I've turned off the automatic login so I always have to type my password when logging in. If something important happens among my friends or family I usually hear about it eventually, even if I miss the Facebook post. That being said, I do check the notifications on most days. From Saturday night to Monday morning I am in monk mode/social media, internet and email detox – not logging in at all. It has been exhilarating. Also, as of writing this, I haven't checked my Twitter account in about six months.

DON'T WATCH THE NEWS

I've learnt that watching the news causes me anxiety over things I can't control. As with Facebook, if something important happens that

I need to know about, I will hear about it. It's a fact of life. I do check a newspaper once or twice a day for headlines. And I stick with papers that are the least hyped up and don't have "news" about the Kardashians.

So, stop complaining that you don't have time and do something about it instead. You will not only improve your health but you will also be more productive and more present with the people you're with, since you won't need to be distracted by thinking ahead. Routines will take care of that for you. Start by doing your time diary, observe your time-management skills, and find out what you can streamline or routinise.

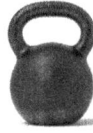

PART 4

Ditch The Excuses

DON'T LET YOUR SUCCESS DEPEND ON WILLPOWER

Picture this: you're excited about your health and fitness routines, and you're motivated to work towards your goals. But the biggest obstacle between you and a fitter, healthier body is your relentless appetite for sweets at work. You are few weeks into your "no sweets" plan and going strong, until that one mad afternoon at work when your stress levels turn your body shades of red. Without warning, you start to entertain the thought of sweet chocolatey goodness. Mmm … Cherry Ripe. You force the evil thought out of your head. But the image of the 16th floor vending machine loaded with chocolate bars floats past your retinas. You slap yourself silly to distract your thoughts. And it works, temporarily.

But no matter how hard you try to ignore it, that devil of a Cherry Ripe crawls back into your mind until it become impossible to resist. You make your way to the 16th floor and make the vending machine sing. But only today, you say. Because tomorrow you will be stronger, more motivated, and even more committed.

And then tomorrow afternoon rolls around. That sexy thing of a Cherry Ripe dances its way back into your mind. You resist for a while but eventually repeat the same familiar cycle and make your way to the 16th floor. And by now your face is red and raw from slapping yourself.

Does this sound familiar? What can we do about it? To find the answer we have to revisit a couple of studies from the past.

Don't think about the polar bear

In his book *59 Seconds: Think a Little, Change a Lot*, Richard Wiseman writes about how Harvard psychologist Daniel Wegner was intrigued by a quote from Dostoevsky's *Winter Notes on Summer Impressions*: "Try to pose yourself this task: not to think of a polar bear, and you will see that the cursed thing will come to mind every minute." Wegner carried out a study and found that this was indeed true – try to ignore a thought and the mind will obsess over it. There have been similar studies since with more of a real-life application. Jennifer Borton and Elizabeth Casey from Hamilton College in New York instructed a group of people to describe the most upsetting thing about themselves. They then told half of the group to suppress the thought for the next 11 days. The rest of the group continued their life as normal. The results showed that the suppression group thought of the negative thing more often during the experiment and rated themselves as more anxious, more depressed and having lower self-esteem. Sounds a lot like what our hero went through with the Cherry Ripe.

Both studies show that pushing a thought out of our heads doesn't work. That's why strict diets where certain foods are labelled "bad" and "off limits" are not the answer. Once something is a "forbidden fruit" it becomes so much harder to resist. Just ask Adam and Eve: the only rule imposed was not to eat the apple. They probably had bananas, pears, blueberries, oranges and avocados to choose from. Yet, label the apple "forbidden" and cast Satan as The Snake, and it became an obsession.

So what chance do you have then? You might be able to fight the urge for a while but unless you have a mind made out of steel, reinforced concrete and barbed wire it is unlikely that you will keep these thoughts out of your head. The snake will tempt you in the shape of a Cherry Ripe.

Relying on willpower just doesn't work.

Reminders of positive benefits

Instead of dwelling on the negatives you wish to remove ("I won't buy a chocolate bar at work"), visualise the positive additions to your life that this habit will introduce ("Snacking on lower GI foods will help me avoid the sugar crash and make me more productive at work"). Remind yourself frequently about the benefits that reaching your goal will bring. Take it a step further and write out a list that you can refer to.

Once you've written the list, place it somewhere you can see it often. If you struggle with mindless eating at work, stick a post-it note on the side of your computer screen. Struggling with mindless eating while watching TV at home? Place the list on your fridge or stick it onto the cupboard door. Frequent reminders are the key.

Steer clear of "forbidden fruits"

As mentioned earlier, it's important to avoid diets where certain food items are off limits. Rather, believe that you can eat whatever you want and not feel guilty about it. One of the many snippets of wisdom I got from reading Georgie Fear's book *Lean Habits For Lifelong Weight Loss* is that having a mindset of "I won't have any now, but I can have a little bit later on" will also go a long away. That way you are not denying yourself anything. Wherever possible, it helps to not have foods at hand that you might have a hard time resisting. That will save you from the willpower fight in the first place. I admit this can be easy at home but a challenge at work ... unless you want to piss off a floor full of colleagues by jamming the vending machine with (low-calorie) chewing gum and super gluing inspirational post-it-notes on it.

Practise mindfulness

Mindfulness is about stopping and taking a moment to notice what is going on in your head. Acknowledge your thoughts, be curious about why you are thinking this way, and accept that this is OK. When you notice an urge to run for the vending machine with coins in your hand, stop for a minute to see what's going on. Maybe you're stressed and anxious and that's your trigger for snacking. Take a moment to acknowledge this stress and anxiety. Is there anything you can do about it? If you can do something to ease the underlying stress that leads to cravings, do it. If there's nothing you can do right now, just acknowledge that you are feeling stressed.

Write down three to five benefits of following a healthier diet

When do you crave certain foods the most? What do you notice about yourself in these moments? e.g. "I notice that I crave Cherry Ripe when I'm stressed."

PLANNING FOR OBSTACLES

Planning strategies to overcome obstacles will dramatically improve your chances of succeeding in life. Major storm heading your way? Better plan an exit strategy or a way to storm-proof the house. Looming nuclear war on the horizon? Better plan an exit strategy or a way to storm-proof the house. Christmas party with the family? Better plan an exit strategy or a way to storm-proof the house. Improving your health is no different. You need a plan. Being successful at reaching your fat-loss target or health goal is about planning in advance how you will act when challenging situations arise. Let's examine a couple of scenarios that you might find yourself in.

1. Walter White as a co-worker

Your co-worker Walter White brings in cupcakes each Wednesday topped with his special blue icing. He's a fantastic cook, the culinary equivalent of John Bonham, and all around top-notch guy. But behind that innocent face sits a mean bastard in the sense of a true food pusher. You try to say no, but often one cupcake turns into three.

2. Hank Moody as a best mate

On Friday afternoons you agree to a couple of drinks with your best mate Hank Moody. But as is often the case with Hank, a couple of drinks turns into a night of debauchery, followed by three quarter-pounders with cheese.

3. Michael Scott as a boss

You often get disturbed by emails from your boss Michael Scott ahead of your planned after-work training session. He truly knows how to waste your time with unproductive, non-urgent tasks. Before you know it, work has taken over and you settle for telling yourself "I'll train later tonight", which doesn't end up happening because of your best mate Hank.

You keep telling yourself next week will be different: you will say no to the cupcakes and Friday night drinks, and you'll get to training no matter what. Then Wednesday rolls around and you end up eating the same three cupcakes. Mr White is persistent. You're held back at work and skip your training sessions. And before you know it, you wake up on Saturday morning covered in French fries and mayonnaise, all Runkled up.

But what if you could take willpower out of the equation? When you make a plan, the need for willpower goes out the window. In *Eating for Life* by Bill Phillips there's this simple exercise:

What are the three biggest obstacles I am going to run into with food?

What are three structures I can put in place to overcome those obstacles?

If food is not your issue but training is, you can use the same template for planning how to get your weekly training sessions in.

Dealing with Walter, Hank and Michael

1. How do you say no to the food-pusher in your life, so that they hear and respect you? Avoid making yourself into a victim by saying "I can't have it". It sounds like someone else is dictating what you can and can't do, as if you have no say in it. Instead, be firm and blunt. A simple "Thank you for offering, but I am not having that today" will suffice. If they keep pushing (most people will, because they feel "threatened" by the odd person out) you can try say something like "I am saving it up for the weekend". A last resort that gets most pushers to stop is and an angry tone and "Can you please stop, I do not want to have any today".

2. How do you keep up a social life without regretting your choices the next morning? This can be tough, and is often the biggest road block for a lot of my clients. Especially if you are attached to binge drinkers and party animals. When I stopped working in bars after a decade, I lost touch with some interesting and fun friends, including some that I were close to up to that point. Simply because getting together always involved big drinking sessions. And it wasn't for me anymore. Not that I was better than others for not binging any more. No, I just wasn't interested in doing it every weekend. I had other interests and frequent hangovers on the couch interfered with what I wanted.

So, my first and best advice that for most people is too blunt and uncomfortable: find new friends whose values match more closely to yours. Another piece of advice: if you are comfortable being semi-sober among a group of intoxicated people, stick with sparkling water and fresh lime. Just get ready to use the anti-food-pusher tactics above. Or hang out with this group when they are not drinking. Try to introduce non-binge drinking activities you can do as a group. Honestly, that's all I've got.

3. How do you manage your time so that work doesn't impinge on your training? Be awesome at your job so the boss allows you to be flexible with your schedule. Block out times for training the same way you would for an important meeting. Convince your employer about the benefits of lunchtime exercise for your work and productivity in the afternoon. The best advice that most people ignore because it's too uncomfortable: get up 90 minutes earlier each morning. Once it's done in the morning it doesn't matter how busy the rest of the day gets.

You may not have a Walter, Hank or Michael in your life – maybe it's Elaine Benes, Peggy Olsen or Rachel Green (with that hair, can you imagine!) Identify your biggest obstacles right now, and come up with structures to overcome them.

What are the three biggest obstacles I am going to run into with food? What are three structures I can put in place to overcome those obstacles?

1.

2.

3.

Best-laid plans

When crafting your plan, planning to simply use your willpower doesn't work. The idea of the plan is that you don't need to rely on willpower at all. You make willpower irrelevant, like the eighth defenseman in hockey.

Whether your goal is to lose five kilograms or run a marathon, you must plan everything step by step. Approach these goals the same way as you would an important project at work. It's unlikely that you'd take on a project without a plan about how to execute it. Solid planning always beats winging it. Trying to lose five kilograms with a vague plan of "training more" won't get you anywhere in the long run. The questions you need to ask are: How much more? How will I fit training in my schedule? If I can't make it to the gym, what is my fall-back plan? How do I keep myself accountable? Is more training the easiest way for me to lose weight or do I have other options?

Let's look at each of those questions and dig a little bit deeper for possible answers.

HOW MUCH MORE AM I GOING TO TRAIN?

Before you scream "AN EXTRA FOUR HOURS A WEEK!" because that's what you think you should say, remember that there is no shame in taking a small first step. As we've already discovered, the first time you fail to maintain the extra four hours a week you will feel like you've failed. That is going to negatively affect your level of motivation.

So what can you do instead? Choose an attainable behavioural goal that you are 90–100% sure you can reach. Maybe it's an hour a week or even 30 minutes. Maybe that's too much and you can only commit to doing 20 bodyweight squats daily. That's cool; it's a start you'll build on.

HOW WILL I FIT TRAINING IN MY SCHEDULE?

So you've decided to do an extra hour each week. What day of the week is the most convenient for you to train? Can you fit in an hour on a single day or is it easier if you do two 30-minute sessions weekly? What time of day is the best for you? If you know that it is very unlikely for you to finish work on time, plan to train in the mornings. That way it is done, and your success doesn't hinge on the ever-unpredictable Michael Scott.

WHAT IF I CAN'T MAKE IT TO THE GYM? WHAT IS MY FALL-BACK PLAN?

The gym may not be the most convenient place for you to train. Maybe it takes too long to get to, and that itself is discouraging. In that case, you could buy some tools such as a TRX and few kettlebells to do your training at home instead.

HOW DO I KEEP MYSELF ACCOUNTABLE?

We've already established that willpower itself will get you nowhere in the long run: you will need more than that. You could find an accountability buddy to keep you in check, someone who you check in with daily or weekly regarding your habit. Talk to one of your friends and ask if they'd be willing to do it for you. Even better, it could be someone working towards a similar goal, so the arrangement is recip-rocal. If a friend is not an option, you can find groups on Facebook. One advantage with social media groups is the support of many individuals going through the same process. Alternatively, you can always hire a trainer to keep you accountable. But don't expect that just because you pay someone money everything will fall in place for you. You still need to work on it.

IS ADDING EXTRA TRAINING THE EASIEST WAY FOR ME TO LOSE WEIGHT? DO I HAVE BETTER OPTIONS?

Whatever your goal, you should spend 80% of your time on actions that give you the greatest return towards your goal. As Josh Hillis writes in *Fat Loss Happens on Monday,* healthy eating is the number one habit for fat loss. If you have to choose between training more or staying at home prepping and cooking meals, choose cooking. That will get you closer to a sustainable fat-loss target than any amount of training ever will. Then spend the remaining 20% of your available time on training and staying active. Always try to get the best bang for your buck. Intelligent training will improve your health in many ways but it isn't the sole solution for fat loss. However, as a cornerstone habit, training can make you more mindful about your eating habits.

As you may have realised by now, all this will take considerably more time than just deciding to lose 10 kilograms, or "get fitter". Most people won't do this planning, and most of them will fail. The people who put in the effort in the beginning will reap the benefits later. They have actionable steps to face the problems that might arise. Be one of *those* people. If you are serious about improving your health, take the time and plan for it.

THE FITNESS EXCITEMENT ROLLER COASTER

Whenever you are about to dive into a new habit it's crucial to understand that it won't be exciting forever. When down the track you feel disheartened, bored and annoyed, remember that 99.9% of folks who start a fitness routine go through these same fluctuations. It's as common as the urge to fart after drinking milk. Yet nobody talks about it because it's not cool.

The initial high … and the first low

As mentioned in the section on motivation, most people new to training, or returning after an extended break, find their fitness journey at least somewhat exciting in the beginning. You have a spring in your step, and you're looking forward to crushing each workout and seeing awesome results. You have "Eye of the tiger" blasting through the headphones. Your social media is littered with *#tabata, #smolov Russian squat program* and *#carrots over beers for Friday night.*

Then the roller coaster swerves sharply downwards. The initial excitement wears off, and you start to dread going to the gym and damn everything it represents.

You might be ready to pull the plug.

But here's a beaming light in a sea of boredom: the lack of excitement will too pass. You'll get excited again. Not quite to the level that you did in the beginning, but excited nevertheless. And since I am sharing secrets, here's one more: that newly found, second wind of excitement will pass too and training will once again become a drag. In fact, I am so sure of it that I drew a diagram. And, I'm sorry if all the curves don't truly reflect how you feel. I am still learning to use Paint.

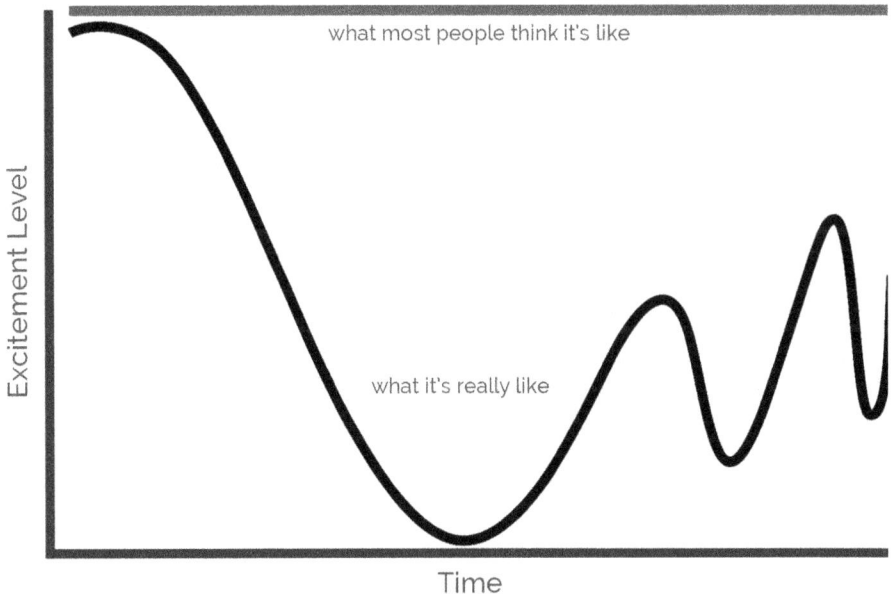

This stuff gets easier over time

Here's the good news. Once you are over the initial hump it gets easier and easier each time. The extremes will become less profound; each up and down a smaller deviation from the norm. It's normal to have periods lacking motivation throughout your training life. Unless you are a robot, training isn't always fun and exciting. Sometimes it's just a thing you do because it's good for you. And it's OK to be as vague as that with your goals during those times. At the times of high motivation you can set bigger and more specific goals.

"Bus bench" and "park bench" training

Strength coach Dan John talks a lot about "bus bench" and "park bench" workouts. Bus bench periods in training are usually short and intense with a specific goal of getting somewhere. Getting ready for a wedding or a beach holiday come to mind. Park bench workouts are what happen throughout the rest of the year. Most of the park bench workouts are medium to low in intensity. They are still done with a goal of improving yourself, but without the rush of getting somewhere. And sometimes they are just done because they have to be done. If all you ever did were park bench workouts with consistency, you'd still be healthier and fitter than the majority, if not all, of the people you know.

Most fitness marketing wants you to believe that training is all about the bus bench: you should always train with the highest intensity, crush weights and eat eggwhites and lifting chalk for breakfast, lunch and dinner. Hardcore training is what sells; it's sexy, exciting and usually sounds amazing: *Neuroblasto Bicepo El'Massivo, Hail The Great Gluteus Maximus Manipulation XXXtreme, Shoulder Shredzoniac Mania 5500 v.2.0.* Not only do the names sound like they could be titles for Spanish erotic novels, often the marketing could be used either way, too.

I used to believe this hype, too. I thought that if I wasn't kicking ass and taking names each session it wasn't worth training. Nobody wants to be told that it's OK not being shredded 365 or just to train for general health. Yawn. Yet the unsexy secret is in showing up on most days and getting something done. Even if it's a shitty training session, you still came in to move. And your long-term health will thank you for it. The few reps you did today might not seem like much. But a few multiplied over a lifetime is a lot of reps.

COMFORT AND HAPPINESS ARE OFTEN INCOMPATIBLE

comfort *n.* a state of physical ease and freedom from pain or constraint

When looking at the definition of "comfort" you'd think that the meaning of life is the eternal search for that very thing. It sounds like the most tranquil place on earth. A place where you get showered with Gummi Bears while watching unicorns play catch with mermaids. Or, failing that, a perpetual state of barbeques and ballgames. But there is such a thing as being too comfortable. Ordering a pizza involves more "comfort" than setting yourself the challenge of learning how to cook. Lounging at home on the couch watching *Seinfeld* is more "comfortable" than joining, and actually frequenting, a gym or sports team. Rarely is long-term happiness achieved this way. Pure comfort without challenges for too long is boring and lacks a certain meaning. What's worse, it can act as fuel for general unhappiness. This doesn't mean that it is a waste of time. Far from it. Holidays, leisure activities and just chilling out are important. But as much as fun as beer, bread, BBQ, ballgames and mermaids are, life would be boring if that's all we ever focused on.

Challenges mean growth

I often wonder why the world's most successful people don't just retire comfortably in the Bahamas but instead keep working and pushing themselves in new directions. Just look at Elon Musk who netted a lazy $165 million for selling PayPal. Then bet it all on building electric cars and, oh I don't know, trying to colonise Mars.

It's because challenges mean growth, and it's hard to grow without being challenged. Even us mere mortals seek growth by signing up for random things that make us uncomfortable. You don't have to colonise Mars to find the thrill of a challenge.

When you try things that you find scary, hard, or maybe even impossible, it brings you a meaningful sense of accomplishment. And if you fail? The only people to ridicule you are those who are suffocated by their own fear.

Stepping outside your health and fitness comfort zone

Seek growth in your health and wellbeing. It's comfortable (and delicious) to stop in for a croissant on the way to work. It's comfortable to order a pizza when you don't feel like cooking. It's comfortable to have a double Baileys on the rocks with a sprinkle of cinnamon when your boss calls you a jackass because the paper you handed in was written in the wrong font. I mean, what's the difference between Calibri and Cambria anyway? But do any of those comfortable actions increase your long-term happiness?

Joining a gym and opening up to a personal trainer about your struggles can be extremely challenging. You might be the strongest performing badass in your professional world, but feel vulnerable when stepping into a gym (or a Zumba class, or a health food store). All I can say is that when you stretch the boundaries of your comfort zone and repeatedly return to it, the new will become the new norm. It's not only your physical health you'll be improving, but also your mental elasticity and strength. Eventually your new activity will become the same as buying calcium-fortified almond milk down at the corner store: not a big deal.

THE STORY YOU TELL YOURSELF MATTERS

"I hate exercise."

"I am a terrible cook."

"I am not a morning person."

"I am a highly-gifted procrastinator."

"My feet pronate. Therefore, I suck at life."

Most of us have a story that we keep telling ourselves. You know you have certain traits, so you keep fitting yourself into the mould you've created, but it's usually a cop-out that stops you from changing the status quo.

I can relate. Once I realised that some of my traits could be explained by being an introvert, I used this as an excuse to not do things that are considered more extroverted. Whenever something felt too uncomfortable and challenging I'd go back to "hey, it's cool, I don't have to do that because I'm an introvert". But I realised the story I was telling myself and the challenges I was avoiding were holding me back. So, I decided to knuckle-punch my self-fulfilling prophecy in the pecker. I was listening to Jason Ferruggia's podcast *Renegade Radio*, and he was talking about improv (acting) classes and how they've helped him. The first time I entertained the idea of improv, my palms were sweating, and I could not have thought of anything more terrifying. Well, unless it involved improv while being in a nest of boa constrictors and Justin Bieber impersonators. But the longer I entertained the idea, the more my desire to try it grew.

Fast forward a year and I am deep into weekly improv classes. Although I am still often uncomfortable in the class, I am much happier doing it than if I had stayed at home picking my nose, wondering if I could. Yes, it was, and still can be, scary and uncomfortable. But more so, it is extremely rewarding because I've shown myself that I *can* do things that I thought I couldn't. Pushing myself there has been thrilling, to say the least. Remember that I am still the guy who a while back could not have thought of anything more terrifying (excluding JB and snakes). I am not telling you this (only) to pump up my own tyres. I am telling this story because if I can get out of my comfort zone and do things that increase my happiness, confidence and sense of self, so can you.

Improve Your Weaknesses and Break Self-Fulfilling Prophecies

I believe that we should work on our weaknesses to become better people. Sure, when it comes to business, work on your strengths and delegate the tasks that are not your strong suit. But when it comes to improving yourself, work on your weaknesses instead of ignoring them, especially if they are causing you to suffer or feel unhappy.

For the next week, try proving yourself wrong. If you think you suck at cooking, start learning more about it while telling yourself "I got this. I am becoming better with practice." If you turn down opportunities to do things early in the morning because you're "not a morning person", try saying "I'm not in the habit of getting up early, but I can try it". Or maybe you are a procrastinator because you've told yourself this for so long. When you get side-tracked you think it's OK because this is just the way you are. And if you keep telling yourself you are too lazy to work out, guess what? You will keep seeking out those habits that lazy people have.

This doesn't mean that you will become a superstar by just believing in it. But you'd be surprised how much you can change by working on your mindset and the habits that you follow.

When I did a habit-coaching course with Omar Ganai from Habitry I learned that the format to start a change is simple:

I want to be good at [insert a task], therefore I need to keep [insert a habit] repeatedly.

Extremely simple, yet frustratingly difficult.

What is your self-fulfilling prophecy that's holding you back? What steps can you take to change it? The only thing holding you back might be your beliefs about the way you are.

A word of caution: some beliefs can be deeply ingrained because of what we have gone through in the past. Please seek professional help if this exercise brings up any trauma or deep-seated issues.

What is the self-fulfilling prophecy I keep telling myself?

BUILDING TRAINING CONSISTENCY

I understand that not everyone is driven by training and lifting goals. For you, each training session might feel like a torture performed by iron, lycra and sweaty butt cracks. You might be in a constant battle between putting your feet up after a long day in the office versus dragging your feet into the gym. The key to unlocking this issue is to build training consistency while still having time to do other things that bring you happiness in life.

Try to remove yourself from your day-to-day thinking and focus on the healthier version of future you. You might even come to enjoy the process; I've seen it happen with most of my clients.

Tell yourself that you are a healthy person. Explain to yourself why you are following a training routine. Reflect on those thoughts.

I picked up this great advice while listening to an episode of the podcast *Bettercast* with Steven Ledbetter and Julie Dirksen. When you are about to skip a workout, drive through the golden arches for dinner, or reach for the third piece of double chocolate brownie, use this future-based thinking to propel you forward, tighten up your shoelaces and pull on your best pair of training shorts. While writing this, I realised that I already picture "future me" when performing a lot of habits in my life, both in and outside of fitness. I do my joint routine each morning because I know that it will make my joints move better and reduce tension around my hips, shoulders and lower back. I don't do it because it's fun, but the thought of how it makes my life better helps me enjoy it somewhat. Future me has the joint mobility of a 30-year-old when I am 75. Same with meditation. On most mornings I would much rather check the NHL trade news than sit on the chair with my eyes closed.

But because I know how it centres me, I keep at it. Future me is calm and collected … with a hint of peppermint and a twist of chamomile.

Be uncompromising with your time

Block time into your schedule for training and treat it as the most important meeting of the week. Don't take other appointments and don't double book. Nothing is important enough to justify cancelling your training. (The only exception is if you or your partner is about to go into labour – you have permission to shuffle the schedule for that. Check to see if the hospital has a gym nearby. Just kidding.) Would I sometimes make more money by shuffling my client sessions around, eating into my own training time? Sure. But I think of it as a choice between money and health. Besides, a healthier and happier coach means healthier and happier clients. When I become overworked, my clients suffer the consequences. And that's not good for anyone.

Quality over quantity

Yes, it's a cliché, but hear me out. You can make great progress by doing 20–30 minutes of quality training a few times a week. What is the most efficient use of your time? If all you can do is a few sets of deadlifts and carries, you are ahead of 99.9% of the population. Heck, you are ahead of the folks who spend hours in the gym doing bicep curls, tricep kicks and ab crunches, among other "exotic" exercises. In a perfect world, you'd be training 45–60 minutes, three days a week, in a fully equipped gym. But, and this is what most new trainees don't understand, it doesn't have to be perfect. Amazing things can happen in 20 minutes if you pour your heart and soul into it – even if all you've got is one kettle-bell at home. For those 20 minutes, all you can do is train: no phones, talking or picking your nose. Just train. Focus on big movements using several muscle groups at the same time. Think swings, goblet squats, carries … Do it properly and you'll be smoked in 14 minutes. Again, quality over quantity. Good attitude for a lot of things in life.

Smarter over harder

The media promotes an all-or-nothing approach to fitness. Embracing a moderate, smart approach is not sexy enough to sell magazines or make exciting television. Entertain this idea for a moment: the next season of *The Biggest Loser* follows Jim who's trying to lose 10 kilograms in 12 months. In the first month, they'll show how he focuses on drinking two glasses of water each day. We'll spy on him via hidden cameras. The cliffhanger moment happens when he's about to head to bed after only having a glass and a half, and then, commercial break! God, the suspense is killing me. Honestly, I would find that fascinating, but I doubt that my opinion reflects that of the typical TV viewer.

There is nothing wrong with being moderate or going easy on yourself. If you are juggling dozens of responsibilities in your life such as kids, relationships and a high-pressure job, the last thing you need is another hard thing to struggle with. If you think you can train twice a week but it might be a stretch, start with one session. If something gives, you can always add a second training session for those weeks. This way, you are always hitting your target and sometimes even exceeding it. How good would that feel compared to deciding to train three times a week but only doing it once? Make your training manageable and you'll have a better shot at sticking with it in the long term. Build confidence that way.

Learn to autoregulate

This is an advanced approach so don't get caught up on this until you have established some of your training habits. Autoregulation means adjusting your training depending on your schedule or how your body feels. Some days or weeks are tougher and some are easier. On busy weeks, you might get to the gym once. During less hectic weeks, you may get in three to four times. When you feel like shit your training session will reflect on it, by design. When you feel great you will make up for it. Learn to ease up when there are too many balls in your court, and they're all on fire. Autoregulation doesn't necessarily work if you don't have a basic training routine in place already. You might have a tendency to skip sessions with the thought of catching up later. Be honest with yourself here.

If autoregulation sounds too confusing for now, this next one works too. I got this idea after reading an article by Alwyn Cosgrove. Basically, he decides on the number of training sessions he's going to do within the next 52 weeks. So let's say you plan on hitting the iron dungeon 100 times within the next 52 weeks. Some weeks you do more, on other weeks you do less, depending on what life throws your way. Write the number on a piece of paper and mark down each time you successfully train. This does not have to be something you do as a New Year's resolution. Just think 52 weeks from today, whether that's January or September. Any time is as good as now. And honestly, now is better than "in the future".

Try a different program

If you've tried weight training a dozen times and you still hate it with the intensity of a thousand burning suns, find a new approach. Have you always trained in the same way? Is it always a similar program? Do you usually start with the same exercises that you end up loathing? Do you stop because you get injured or don't know how to do an exercise? Try something completely new. A different plan, a new set of exercises, a different gym. What if for the next four weeks all you do is a 30-minute walk with a heavy backpack, two or three days a week?

And when you do actually skip a workout, you haven't fallen off the wagon. Fitness isn't even a wagon. It's a slow-moving, never-ending row of carriages and you can jump on anytime you want. It is always going and every day of your life you can decide "here we go!" and hop on.* But to give you a bit of urgency, the longer you travel on the fitness train the further you'll probably go in life, both in quality and quantity.

*I read this somewhere but can't remember where or by whom. Great advice.

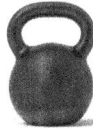

PART 5

Find Your Definition Of Fitness

HOW DO YOU DEFINE FITNESS?

All of us should have our own definition of what we want out of our training plan, eating habits and the lifestyle that we've chosen. Your definition of fitness shouldn't be influenced by what Marcus down the road, or Silvia on Instagram holds important, but what matters the most to you. Once you have a clear map of what health and fitness means to you, it's easier to navigate through the trends, gimmicks, celebrity diets and other junk that gets thrown in your face each time you turn on a television or open a magazine or internet browser. The definition will do wonders for your odds of reaching your goals.

When you can articulate what being "fit" means to you, you can make decisions based on that definition. You can avoid guilt when you make food choices that others might consider "unhealthy", or when you opt for a walk with a friend instead of smelling the butt sweat at your local gym, because you know that these decisions are leading you towards your goals.

For some the definition of fitness is being strong enough to lift a car and sporting a neck that risks them getting locked in a church belltower. For some it's about being fit enough to jog to the bus stop, cook delicious (and not always ultra-healthy) meals for the family while keeping their weight under control, or not feeling bad about taking a bottle of wine to a picnic. And for me? It's about using healthy lifestyle habits to improve my longevity and quality of life as I get older. Not do things today that will have a major negative impact on those qualities tomorrow. But at the same time doing it without making me miserable today. It's a fine balance and I don't nail it every single day. But most days I am close enough. And that's exactly what fitness is for me. Today, anyway. Ask me again in a year and I might have changed my mind.

Write down your definition of health and fitness

SET YOUR OWN STANDARDS FOR A PERFECT BODY

Western society is obsessed over six-packs, big arms, thigh gaps and firm butts. I get that most of those qualities (I never understood the appeal of a thigh gap) are aesthetically pleasing for the eye, and I'm not above that. But I look at aesthetically pleasing bodies differently because I know what sort of sacrifices they are made from. With physique, we eventually hit a point when the returns of investment don't match the input. And when I see someone sporting an out-of-this-world physique I can't help but wonder about all the amazing things they could be pouring their time into instead. And again, just to limit some of the hate-mail I'm bound to receive, I'm not talking about people who have to look a certain way because of their job, such as modelling, or because they do it for a sport, such as bodybuilding. (While I can't wrap my head around bodybuilding as a sport, I put its practitioners in the same category as any athlete who needs to spend a great deal of time to get to the top in their chosen field.) But for any of you whose success in life doesn't depend on how good you look in a bikini or a tight pair of trunks when getting out of turquoise water: if you train and focus on getting stronger, moving better and being pain-free, are not overweight and have health markers in the top end of the "ideal" range, you are fine. Trust me. You are 90% there and most likely look fitter than most of the people on this planet. But to me, spending enormous amounts of time, money and resources to get that last 10% is borderline insanity. I know, because I've been there. Chasing that 10% might be what brings your health markers down. Why not pour all those resources into something that actually has meaning? Mesmerise people by learning to juggle, feed the homeless, or go pat abandoned cats in the shelter.

Being a trainer, it was easy to live in this illusion where everyone trains all the time, obsesses over their looks and is interested in how much weight they just lifted. Everyone on the outside of the bubble looked weird. Why are others not investing as much time into their looks? Don't they get it? Once I took a step back, I realised that what we do is not normal. Most people don't actually live this way. Most people don't train five to seven days a week or worry about how many calories they just ate. Most people don't stress about how that extra beer is going to affect their bench press next week. And if we look beyond the Western society and societies impregnated by Western values, training purely for looks (beyond a certain point) is almost absurd.

Validating our self-worth

Maybe someone's already researched this and made a conclusion, but here's my hypothesis: we put so much effort and energy into "perfecting" our bodies because we are lacking a bigger purpose in life. We are lost, so we grab onto anything that gives our existence meaning, no matter how shallow and artificial that action might be. We lack courage and strength to be ourselves so we look for acceptance from our "friends" on social media or compliments at the dinner table. We hide our insecurities behind a mask of pumped muscle, shredded abs and breast augmentations. Look around you: observe people who are extremely confident, charismatic and seemingly comfortable being themselves. How about Richard Branson, Johnny Depp, Michelle Obama, Jay-Z? Do they spend excessive amounts of time in gyms to achieve a perfect physique? Obviously I have no inside information into their routines, but just by judging a book by its cover, I doubt they spend countless of hours in gyms. Probably just enough to be healthy. And they all look great in their own way. How they look is just a complement to time well spent elsewhere.

Even the greatest bodybuilder of all time, Arnold Schwarzenegger, looked just like a normal person while he was the governor of California. Not bad, not unhealthy, just a slightly more muscular version of an average 60-year-old man. Maybe that was because he had a bigger purpose in life than to pump weights. Now, as he is acting in movies again, he is jacked out of his mind because it goes hand in hand with his purpose: looking good on screen. But that's not the purpose of an average man in his 60s.

We all need to take a step back and realise what's important in life. Is it having a six-pack, or is that just what we've been made to believe? We see "perfect" bodies on TV shows, magazine covers and catwalks. They become part of our reality. You might think that you're less of a person if you look normal instead of sizzling and dripping with sexiness. Hey, I thought that, too. Luckily, I stopped moments before the breast augmentation part. In all seriousness though, I still occasionally struggle with trying to fit into the mould that is forced upon me as a male in the fitness industry: that I am not muscular enough or my shoulders are not broad enough. We all have our insecurities, and it's normal. Just because others think a certain look is the pinnacle of perfection doesn't mean that you have to strive to look like that. Set your own goals and targets, accept them and be content when you get there. Hell, maybe you're there already.

Am I contradicting myself here? Does this mean that what I do for work is meaningless? After all, I help people with training, fitness and health. No, far from it. I'm proud of the fact that I help people to have healthy, resilient bodies so they can do awesome things outside of the gym. I don't want anyone to become a gym-rat because they read my book.

DON'T CONFUSE HEALTH AND FITNESS GOALS

I want to help you to be clear on your goals and to understand what is possible and what's not. Setting the right expectations is key in avoiding disappointment. Here's a common scenario I often explain to new clients. For a second, imagine that you're sitting next to me for a goal-setting session.

After 15 minutes of talking about our mutual fascination of World War II memorabilia, we are finally discussing your goals. You want to be healthier, feel better and drop some of the belly fat that's crept up over the last few years. You'd also like to ease some of that low back soreness you're getting. That's cool; we can work on that.

Here's how we would approach it. Start by eating a bit more protein and vegetables while reducing the intake of food that comes in a cardboard box. Let's include some resistance training with a plan of progressively getting stronger. We make an effort to not resort to only doing high-intensity, low-resistance, high-volume bunny-rabbit types of training. For the back pain, assuming that a more serious prognosis is cleared by a clinician, we'll start by looking at your movement patterns. Maybe I need to refer you out, maybe I don't.

Well, that wasn't too difficult.

But then, to my bewilderment, you throw a deep left hook to the jawbone. As we get a bit further into our chat you bring up how you'd also like to run a marathon under 4:20, get a six-pack à la Terry Crews and sport a pair of thick guns hanging off your shoulders where your arms are currently located. Although I admire your ambition, you might not realise it but we are dealing with two sets of goals that don't necessarily go together. The first set of goals you mentioned (to feel better, be healthier, drop fat, reduce back pain...) are health-focused, while the second set of goals (marathon, TC six-pack, build enormous arms) falls into the fitness goals category.

Why does it matter that the goals are from different categories? Because you can be extremely fit while at the same being extremely unhealthy. It's like wanting to play in the NRL (or NFL) for the pending health benefits that participation in collision sport brings. Think of the concussions, broken bones and stiff upper lips. It's rare to find a competitive sport that wouldn't somehow ask you to trade health for fitness and performance. Even darts players can develop elbow and wrist tendinitis from too much throwing. Now, now, contain your laughter.

There is nothing wrong with this trade-off but it often gets overlooked. Sure, you can work on injury prevention (a fancy term that often just means "don't train like a arsehole") but when you chase performance, your health will usually take a backseat. It's impossible to be on top of them both at the same time. You can still push performance goals at the gym, which involves things like getting to your first (or 10th) pull-up, push-up or mastering the get-up. This is about you improving yourself. But if you keep reaching higher and further, at some point you'll have to ask yourself whether goal of 30 pull-ups or a 48 kg get-up is worth the risk. As soon as you turn training into competition against others or let your ego take over, you will risk trading health for fitness. I've done both and been reminded of this many times in the past.

So, if you train for a competition or for a fitness goal, have at it. The possible achievement could well be worth the sacrifices that you'll have to make. Just acknowledge it all in advance. But don't miss out on life because you sacrificed health to break the record of "human get-up" (a get-up holding a live person, although dead would be even harder) only to get your name on top of the scoreboard at your local gym. In a year's time no-one will remember it. But you will have to live with the possible negative consequences of torn shoulder ligaments and stiff upper lip for the rest of your life. Not to mention the consequences of finding a dead person in the first place. What were you thinking?

Your training should help you to become better at another task, whether it's for a sport or to improve the quality of your daily life outside the gym. Once the training itself becomes the end goal, you will start to run into trouble and possible injuries. Another piece of wisdom from Dan John: If your goal is to be healthy, think of training as something that you do for tomorrow, so that you'll be able to do the activities that you want to do in life. This is not to say you can't train hard; you can and you absolutely should, occasionally. Just keep the end goal in mind.

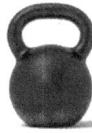

PART 6

Training Rules For Adults

YOU DON'T NEED TO TRAIN LIKE AN ATHLETE

Fitness shouldn't be something that makes you miserable. You might think that to get anywhere with your training you need to keep adding weight to the bar, squeeze out a couple more reps, or only squat ass-to-grass. "Eat clean and train like an athlete" is commonly dispelled advice. You might believe that you can cheat on Saturdays but otherwise your calories have to be spot on and every macronutrient has to have its place in the diet. Earn the "bad" foods! Your body's a temple! Otherwise, why do you bother showing up in the first place?

No. Fitness should add positive energy, productivity, happiness and joy to your life. If you fit into any of the following categories, you *shouldn't* train and eat like an athlete:

- You have a job that requires you to get shit done in order to get paid.

- You have a family that needs you.

- You have friends that mean a lot to you.

➲ You have pets that want your attention.

➲ You have a hobby that you enjoy.

➲ You have a partner who deserves some of your time.

Now, if you happen to fit in any of these following categories, you *should* train and eat like an athlete:

➲ You are an athlete who competes in athletic endeavours.

➲ You are a movie star or model whose work requires your body to be in an athlete-like state.

If you are not an athlete but live in your parents' basement, and don't pay rent or cook your own food, you shouldn't brag about how hardcore your life in the gym is and how everyone else is weak and full of excuses. You shouldn't tell people that to get there you just have to want it hard enough. It doesn't work like that once you are in the real world where mum's not cooking you meatballs.

The saying "train like an athlete" sets unrealistic expectations of what you should be capable of when you most likely have things in your life that should always take priority over training. If your important relationships, work or health suffer because you train like an athlete, your life is out of balance. If any of these suffer because you have to always eat "clean" (a term I absolutely loath) or hit the iron dungeon, your life is out of balance.

There are times when you are allowed to squat the same amount of weight that you did before. You don't have to add more reps, more weight or go harder in any way. If your program takes 60 minutes but you only have 15, it's OK to do the absolute minimum. If you are not an athlete, you are still winning by showing up and moving.

Don't let anyone tell you that you *need* to do something. Sure, others can give you ideas, and encourage you to try something new, uncomfortable or challenging. But don't let others force their ideals onto you. You get to decide what you want. Whatever you do, do not look up to the ultra-fit trainer who has a 14-pack as a prime example of what is possible. Don't even look up to him for inspiration. Because us trainers and coaches spend our days in a gym, moving around, exploring and experimenting. That's our job. Most of us do it because we love it. But you don't have to be passionate about it the same way as we are. Nor should we expect you to be. Also, as a side note, having a 14-pack is not a definition of health or success in life.

As long as you move well and do it often, eat healthy more often than not, wear a seatbelt, don't do heroin, avoid the pink grapefruit juice cleanses, and have all your other health markers in check (blood pressure and weight come to mind) you're doing well. And if you can keep those up while doing the things that make you happy, you are winning. Sure, I'd love it if everyone was as excited about overhead pressing and eating sauerkraut as I am. Yet I acknowledge that is not the case for most people. And I too go through phases of not giving a flying shit about any of it. For most people good enough is, well, good enough. It doesn't have to be perfect. If Suzie shows up for her training session 10 minutes late after a terrible day at work, and one hour of sleep because her one-year-old son was screaming his head off, she doesn't need me to make her feel awful about coming in late. She doesn't need me to push her to go heavier on the weights or to hit the new record on prowler sprints. And the last thing she needs is me to question why she didn't eat any protein for breakfast. Most likely any of those things will only make her feel worse. Against all those odds, Suzie showed up to move anyway (even if she is only going through the motions and yawning at me while doing so). She doesn't want to talk about macros, micros, the level of oxygen in water or the antioxidants in blueberries. And that's fine. In my book, she is still winning.

Of course, there will always be people who love being pushed and love to keep reaching for their personal best every single time. And that's great; have at it. I'll support you all the way. But being healthy doesn't mean sacrificing the other aspects of life. It's not about being perfect. When you are at 90–95%, that is good enough. That last 5–10% is where the shit starts to hit the fan, big time. The wrong things will take priority.

Fitness has to fit into your life, not the other way around. Don't mess up the wheel by putting too much emphasis on a single spoke.

What do you actually need?

Since you are looking at yourself from the inside you might miss the bigger picture. This is a tough question to answer by yourself. It's easy to get overwhelmed when stepping into a gym: there are rows of machines to choose from, kettlebells, barbells, dumbbells, bands, benches, suspension trainers, balls, walls and chin-up bars. The list reads like the inventory of your local hardware store. And then there's the mysterious thing in the corner ... the one that looks like a medieval sorcerer's torture device.

And no matter how hard you try, it's difficult to not be biased towards a certain style of training.

The first problem with a typical gym-goer

A typical gym-goer, in a corporate world such as where I work, has a sedentary office job that involves eight hours of hunched-over sitting every day. An hour before and after work is spent commuting, for a total of two hours or so. Then the day is capped off with three hours of sitting watching the television at night. Do you think what these folks need is to sit on exercise equipment, or do ab crunches, only to get more hunched?

No. They need the opposite: to get out of the hunched position. The body is meant to move. You are meant to do things while moving: squat, press, pick things off the ground, carry stuff around, roll and crawl on the floor. If we ignore this for long enough, the body will forget these crucial movement patterns and the brain will start pruning itself by reducing neural connections. When we are not using certain movements frequently enough, the brain thinks the movements are not necessary for us to keep. Over time, this leads to poor movement quality and accelerated ageing. The Tinman's movement flow will end up looking smooth compared to ours.

The solution is to build our training around squatting, hinging, pulling, pushing, jumping, throwing, slamming, carrying and crawling. And if you've never done any of that, don't jump (pun intended) straight into the deep end. Rather, progress to get there slowly.

The second problem with a typical gym-goer

I don't like to generalise, but I will anyway: most guys want to lift heavy weights and bench six days a week (the seventh is arms) when what they really need is some additional mobility work sprinkled with some conditioning. This doesn't mean that guys need to stop benching. Just balance it out with other stuff. Who knows, the numbers in bench might even go up as a result.

Since I've started, allow me to keep generalising. Most of the ladies could use some heavier strength work to complement the yoga, Pilates, cardio, or the usual sets of tricep kickbacks-to-death. This doesn't mean stopping yoga or Pilates, but adding a bit of variety. If you only do one type of training over time, one thing is guaranteed to happen: your body will reach a breaking point. Too much lifting without mobility is no bueno. Too much yoga without lifting is no bueno. Too much of any single activity throws you off balance. Unless your goal is to have the biggest squat in the southern hemisphere or to be part of the Cirque du Soleil's flexibility act, you will be better off adding variety to your training.

I love pressing heavy, banging out chin-ups and general panting while lugging heavy stuff around. I love it because, although I am not exactly Herculean, I am good at it. What I don't like is mobility work and all sorts of nitty-gritty corrective work. I don't like it because I suck at it. It's a hit on my ego every single time. Yet at the same time I desperately need it.

So here's how you solve this question: you need to do what you find annoyingly hard to do. In order to have a well-rounded, pain-free body, you need to do stuff that you suck at.

Knowing when to stop

Our world is plagued with the mindset of more: sacrificing sleep to work more hours, making more money to buy more space. Buying more stuff to fill up the big, empty space. Yet, owning more shit doesn't equal a better life. It just means owning more shit. We have the same "more is better" mindset with exercise too. But more is not better: better is better. If exercising hurts, or if you are sick and run down, it's your body telling you to either stop or to slow down. It's a safety mechanism to protect the body. It's not "weakness leaving the body", or "no pain no gain". It's the warning light that says, "Slow the fuck down because your wheels are coming off!"

We ignore sustainable plans that proclaim that a little over a long time is the secret sauce, the almighty magic button. Nah, it sounds too simple, and most definitely not hardcore enough. No, let's attack fat loss by adding more exercise with higher intensity so we can feel tired and as if we've accomplished something.

Instead of measuring success in the gym by the amount of sweat that you can expel from your body, focus on asking one question: "Did I get better today?" Usually after finishing your training session you should feel like you could repeat the session in a few hours. If 12 hours later you are still hyperventilating into a paper bag, seeing small green men dancing on the horizon, and need an IV drip of Gatorade to function, you've probably done too much. Walk away like you could do more. Leave room for tomorrow. Training is not a war. It is just training. The gym should be a place where you predominantly go to improve yourself. You go there so you can squeeze more out of life outside of the gym. Strength and conditioning specialist Brett Jones describes strength as a bucket. The bigger your bucket the more stuff your body can do. And it works with fitness too, your goal is to own a bigger bucket so you can fill it with more life experiences. But most people seem to train to get better at training. Somehow we've turned gyms into sweat fests where people come to exercise, or rather exorcise, their demons by doing more, more and more. If one high-intensity workout a week is good, then 10 must bring you to the god-level.

We've lost the mind–body connection with training. Instead of asking "How does this weight feel when I press it over my head?", we're just counting the next rep, and the next rep, and the next to get to the end of it. We've lost the art and appreciation of graceful movement, the focus on how a movement feels. In martial arts and yoga this connection still exists. But in fitness we rely on technology to tell us whether we trained hard enough, walked far enough or burned enough calories. Although I struggle to associate myself with bodybuilding, even Arnold said in the 70s (watch *Pumping Iron*) that with each rep he focuses on how the muscle *feels* when the weight is lifted. Somehow, somewhere, we took a wrong turn.

What's on the line for you?

I know how it feels when you have to step back and take time off from training or not go as hard as you used to. I've trained through pain too many times. Not because I am tougher than the rest, but because I was dumber than the rest. I ended up with a torn labrum in the shoulder, golfer's elbow, low back pain, neck pain, and knee tendonitis. I let these get worse and worse while not looking after myself. The end result was always the same: forced rest for longer than I'd like to admit. So trust me when I say that I get it. Modifying training because something doesn't feel like it should is frustrating. But modifying is better than forced rest after tearing your shoulder out of its socket, or escalating your cough to pneumonia. You'll not only miss months of training, but also have a poorer quality of life outside of the gym. I mean, playing frisbee golf with your throwing arm in a sling is only fun for those watching you trying to throw with your non-dominant arm.

There's an amazing power in being in tune with your body. My challenge for you is to not train to the point of fatigue and injury. Get stronger, improve your movement. And yes, work hard and still challenge yourself, but finish fresh. After each month, reassess how your body feels.

When the goal is to improve how your body looks and feels

If you are training for overall fitness, a.k.a. general fitness, a.k.a. total fitness (meaning you want to get stronger, drop a bit of fat, stay lean and release stress) there are no strict rules on how to structure your training routine. If you have no desire to compete in powerlifting, why work up to a massive deadlift, squat or bench press? If you are not looking to take part in any body-composition competitions, why go on mad, unsustainable diets? You can do both if that's what *you* want, but don't let someone tell you that there is only one way for you to train or to eat. A trainer who says that all their clients have to squat, bench and deadlift because "it's the best way" is putting you into a training mould that they have created for themselves, instead of moulding the training to suit you. It's the same if a trainer gives a general cookie-cutter diet to all their clients. It might work brilliantly for Person B while at the same time being catastrophic for Person A. If you are Person A, it might make you feel like a failure and lose your motivation for any future effort. Imagine if that was the one chance you were willing to give to change your lifestyle, and it all crumbled because you were not met at your starting point.

I agree that everyone should know how to squat, hinge and push, but these can be achieved in more ways than just by doing barbell lifts. Not everyone has to put a barbell on their back or deadlift from the floor, nor is it the best way to go about training for everyone. I won't get anyone even smelling the bench press until they can do 10 solid push-ups. Most of the time we won't go there even after that, unless that's what *the client* wants to be good at.

For you, Jane or Joe (and I include myself in here as well since I am not competing in anything, except for trying to be generally awesome), the best way to get to your general health goal is to do so with patience. By focusing on compound, multi-joint movements, you can realise your long-term health goals without ever touching a barbell if you don't want to. You can realise your long-term body composition goals without ever counting calories or going on a strict diet. And as much as I like to promote resistance training for health benefits beyond the looks, the best way to improve your health is to choose an activity that you can do with consistency over time. For some it might mean lifting weights and for others it might be mountain biking. As long as you stick to it and do it safely, it doesn't matter. And if you want to alternate by shifting from mountain biking to weights and onto badminton, it's all good. Do what *you* enjoy, as long as it improves your overall health and fitness.

Keep in mind that as you get closer to your capacity you will start seeing diminishing returns. This means that at some point you will have to put in a lot of work while seeing very little progress. When you are working closer to your capacity, your risk of injury will increase. And if you are not planning to compete in your chosen activity, I don't see the benefit of this. You are risking your health to feed your ego, in order to achieve some number that in the end means nothing (unless, again, this is what *you* want and it keeps you coming back to training).

When you are training for overall health you can be flexible with structuring your training. Maybe one month you focus on perfecting the get-up. Then the next month you focus on bodyweight training. Maybe the following month you want to practise your squat, before moving onto something completely different again. As long as you are generally getting better in how your body feels and, *gasp!,* looks, I don't care what you want to do – as long as you go about it safely.

IMPROVE YOUR FITNESS BY IMPROVING YOUR MOVEMENT

The goal of this chapter is not to scare you into stopping your fitness efforts. Quite the opposite: the goal is to get you wondering if you could do better. If you are a novice to training or contemplating starting, let me tell you this: too often, a timid person finally musters the courage to start a fitness program, does something that is beyond their capability, gets injured, and never sets their foot in the gym again. It's a tragedy. Whether you are a seasoned trainee or a novice, working on your movement quality will help to take the brakes off so you can accomplish your goals not only more safely, but also faster.

As we've discussed, the only way most trainees know how to measure the "success" of a training session is whether they are gassed (exhausted) at the end of it. The closer we are to coughing up blood after a high-intensity workout, the more success we've achieved. It's one of the reasons why we, the training population, have more musculoskeletal injuries than the non-training population. We take on fitness to become healthier, yet achieve the opposite. And we keep coming back and doing it over again. That is ignorance and idiocy at its finest.

Prioritise movement quality

Most trainees are too focused on the fitness side of things and completely ignore their movement quality. And I get it. If you are conditioned to use your level of tiredness and soreness (both of which are fallacies) as a measuring stick for success, it can be frustrating to take a step back from intense training. It will feel like you are not going anywhere. But to have long-term success in training, movement quality has to come first.

To illustrate this point, we have talk about aeroplanes. You can't improve the engine turbines of a Boeing 747 without improving the frame, the wheels, and everything in-between. The best-case scenario when only improving the turbines is that the 747's original frame will limit the capabilities of the more powerful engine. The plane won't fly any faster despite all the money and man-hours involved. The weak links will hold back the plane's performance. This is equivalent to you wasting countless hours in the gym, wondering why you aren't getting results: you're trying to load fitness onto a body that can't make the most out of it. Your frame is limiting what the engine can do. The worst-case scenario of only improving the turbines is that the powerful 747 engines will rip the original frame into pieces during take-off. In the gym, this means injuries, missed training sessions, declining results and everything that follows forced rest. And sadly, that is what I see all the time. As a matter of fact, someone, somewhere in the world at this very moment is committing this. It is especially true of men who are trying to impress *ze ladiez* (or other men) with magnificent feats of strength. I also see women with poor-quality movement jump into high-intensity programs and classes that are beyond their current capabilities. It's a shit-storm in the making. Your movement quality is the springboard for everything you want to get better at in or outside of the gym. There's wisdom (and safety, and pending future awesomeness) in mastering the basics first. Yet, it is unpopular because it requires long-term thinking and an abundance of patience.

Know and improve your movement baseline

I am in favour of a yearly "movement screen" for everybody, an idea I believe I first heard on the *Ask Mike Reinold* podcast. It would be just like a check-up at your dentist or doctor. The dentist tells you what work your teeth need and whether you have to be more diligent with your mouth hygiene – possibly reaching behind that far left back tooth more often. The doctor will tell you about your blood work and whether there are preventative measures you should take. Your movement specialist would tell you what you need to work on. If you spend your days slaving away in a cubicle, it would likely be things such as upper back and hip mobility. Not only would this be a preventative measure to avoid pains and aches that come with poor movement quality, but it would also get you better results. Working on movement quality is like putting money in the savings account for the future – to help you keep more independent as you get older. Use it or lose it, as the old folks say.

If you are new to training, make sure to get your movement screened first. A good place to start is the *Functional Movement Systems* website to find a person certified in the Functional Movement Screen. If you've been training for a while, keep checking your movement baseline.

Don't let your fitness efforts negatively affect your movement quality, but learn to improve and maintain both.

FOCUS ON MOVEMENT GOALS TO IMPROVE HOW YOU LOOK

For most people, their first introduction to exercise is all about losing weight or keeping the weight off. Combating our sedentary lifestyle and the weight gain that comes with it is one of the biggest problems our society is facing today. It's a growing issue, and it's not going away with the tactics we are currently using. So, I propose a little shift in attitude towards training. First off, we shouldn't think of training as something that we *have* to do. We shouldn't treat it as a punishment for our unhealthy food choices. As long as we keep doing that, we put a negative spin onto something that really is a privilege. We get to move our bodies and explore the world around us while doing it. How amazing is that!

I've missed a chance of working with a client because I wasn't willing to put them through the latest gut-wrenching, head-exploding, high-intensity workout that they saw on TV or in a magazine. I've lost clients because at the end of their session they were disappointed they weren't spitting a kidney out on the gym floor. Everyone wants to do the most advanced training from the get go. It's sometimes hard and confusing to realise that there are steps that you have to take. You have to earn the right to do more advanced movements. It's like me going to medical school and asking to do a surgery on a baby the first day because it looked cool on *Grey's Anatomy*.

You gotta earn it

I like to use the Functional Movement Systems tagline "First move well, then move often". As with anything in life, we are drawn to the cool stuff instead of learning how to do the basics first. But you have to earn the right to do advanced workouts. You skip enough steps and they will come and bite you in the ass later on. If you skip learning how to hinge and squat with your own bodyweight first, you haven't earned the right to touch a weight. This may sound harsh, but I've been there, and it has gotten me injured. That's why I now preach movement integrity.

You wouldn't trust a pilot who skipped the landing training in school so they could get to the cockpit of a 747 sooner. Why would you trust a body that hasn't learned the skills of quality movement? Slow and steady might not sound exciting, but over the long term you will breeze by the folk who ran themselves into the ground early on. And trust me, learning the basics is a challenge in itself. It just doesn't make cool Instagram stories.

Training to build independence

The only goal of any training program should be to make you better at other tasks in life. It should improve how you move outside of the gym. Don't make the fitness your end goal. When I saw physical therapist Gray Cook speak at the Long Beach Perform Better Seminar in 2016, he said it better than I ever could:

The goal is to work towards balance, independence and sustainability. Most fitness programs target quantity over quality, progress over protection, opinions over expertise and evidence, unsustainable over sustainable, dependent over independent.

Instead of looking at your training through the fat-loss filter, you could look at it as a way of building more independence. The more thought-out and frequent your movement plan is, the bigger your base, a.k.a. independence, will be. If your training goals are to become more mobile, agile, and pain-free, all the while getting stronger, you will have a bigger base. You will keep your independence for longer. And what usually comes with a frequent movement practice and increased independence is fat loss. When you are not overweight, you will be able to move better. And the better you can move, the more independence you will have. Your joints will hurt less because you are carrying less weight. The less excess weight you carry, the better you will move, the more independence you will have, and the better you will feel. It's a systemic cycle of awesomeness. Hear that? That's your head. It just exploded.

Focusing on movement goals

As boring as it sounds, "training for tomorrow" is one of the best goals you can have. By focusing on improving yourself for tomorrow, you will naturally focus on the following:

- Body composition. The less fat you carry (to a point), the healthier you can be.

- Strength. It will make most things in life easier. You are more capable of doing things. And stuff.

- Power. As you grow older, power will deteriorate 1.5 times faster than strength. "Power" can be something as simple as being able to catch your balance when you are about to fall in the shower. Or as complicated as doing back flips on your skis.

⊙ Mobility. If you are in pain and not moving well, you are not really getting the most out of tomorrow. If you don't use it today, you'll lose it tomorrow.

Sure, there are times when you'll want to focus on one of these aspects more than the others. Strength is a good example: maybe you want to build up to a heavy get-up or break your deadlift record. You pursue your strength goal while doing the minimum to maintain the others. Over time, you should cycle through all four aspects of training to keep things in balance. And during busy times, you can just do the minimum to maintain all of them without trying to build on any. That's cool too.

Master the three big "ups"

So if independence equals fat loss, what kind of training should you do to build independence? This is so simple, yet, again, not easy. You'll achieve independence by mastering humble bodyweight exercises, as they require the most control. You can't rely on outside resistance for stability – you have to create it yourself. Instead of focusing on the number on the scale, let's focus on these big three 'ups'.

You can access the video demonstrations for these exercise and the required mobility tests at **RepsAndTheRest.com/SpandexNotCompulsory**

The get-up

The get-up requires strength, stability and mobility as well as a Zen-like focus.

Goal: 1 × get-up each side with a shoe balanced on your fist.

How to build to a get-up:

1. Check you've got the required mobility to get your hips and shoulders into the positions they need to go. Using the functional movement screen, in a shoulder mobility test, your fists need to be within 1.5 times your hand length from each other. In an active straight-leg raise, the ankle should clear the opposite knee. You should also be able to roll from your back to stomach using just your upper body.

2. Break the get-up into parts focusing on the roll, reach, tabletop, sweep, half-kneel, and standing, hammering each sequence until you are ready to progress. Don't rush this exercise.

Side note 1: It's as much about the arm that is on the ground as it is about the arm holding the cup, the shoe or the kettlebell.

Side note 2: Let your skill, not your ego, guide your limits.

The push-up

One of the most underutilised, and, oh, so frequently butchered exercises. And, no, you are not too advanced for it. This will tell us more about your body than you might think. A proper push-up requires tension throughout the entire body, something that is not familiar to most gym-goers.

I train the general population and I value this exercise more than I value the bench press.

Goal:

- 30 × push-ups (or more) for men at their prime. As you get older, this number will start to decline (unless you're a badass).

⊙ 10 × push-ups (or more) for women at their prime. There's no "girl" push-ups. That term makes me want to run head-first into a jungle of swinging axes. And lions. Who are also swinging. While holding an axe.

How to build to a push-up:

You don't have to be able to do a full push-up right out of the gate. Here's a progression format that I use successfully with my clients.

1. Check you've got the required wrist control. Your active wrist extension should be at least 80 degrees.

2. High tension plank × 10 breaths. If this is too hard, you might have to work on bracing and tension. Think of pushing the floor away from you, closing a zipper on your knees, bring belt buckle to belly button, isometrically pull hands towards toes, make a double chin. Breath.

3. Elevated push-ups. Elevate your hands high enough so you can do three sets of five push-ups. This could be on a box or even against a wall. Once you can do 3×5, move to a lower box.

4. Negative push-ups and isometric holds at the bottom position. This is a good tool to use if you struggle to drop low enough when on the ground and tend to do "Bondi" push-ups (half-assed and ego-driven).

5. Full push-ups. The secret to getting more and more reps out is to practise the exercise frequently without tiring yourself by going to failure. Finish each set while still feeling fresh. I recommend looking up Pavel Tsatsouline's *Fighter Pull Up Program* and using the same princi-ples for push-ups.

And if you are a woman, notice how there's no such thing as "female", "girly" or "kneeling" push-ups. Because these terms are shit. As a woman you should be able to ace the full push-ups. And when you do, that's *the* shit.

Start at the level you're currently at. Once you've cleared that level, you can progress to the next. Don't skip steps, as it will come to haunt you later.

The chin-up

Again, this exercise requires more than just strong pulling. You must be able to stabilise through your entire body. And, no, you can't train this while sitting on the lat pull-down machine.

Goal:

- 10 × chin-ups for men, but 15 if you're badass. Which you obviously are since you are reading this book.

- 3 × chin-ups for women, but do 10 and you are in an extremely rare group of badasses. Which you obviously are since you are reading this book.

How to build to a chin-up:

This is often a longer process than the push-up. Don't get discouraged along the way.

1. The required movement screens before giving into the temptations of chin-ups: back to wall shoulder flexion with core control, keeping ribs to hips and avoiding excessive arch through the back. Then,

standing overhead scapular retractions, to show that you can control your shoulder blades when your arms are above the head.

2. As with the push-up, high-tension plank × 10 breaths.

3. Hanging scapula retractions, to show you can control your shoulder blades in a hanging position.

4. TRX rows, to show that you can row with core control, three sets of five with your body parallel to the ground. If you don't have the shoulder mobility to go overhead (or can't control your shoulder blades overhead), this is where you'll stay until the movement screens are cleared.

5. Isometric and negative chin-up holds. Not going to failure and doing these frequently are the keys to success here. Occasionally try to do a full one from the bottom to see where you get stuck. Then use that point as a mark where you do the isometric holds. I've recently started teaching these on rings as the set up is easier.

6. Chin-up. Woooohoooo! As with push-ups, the secret to getting more and more reps out is to practise the movement frequently without tiring yourself by going to failure. Finish each set while still feeling fresh. Again, check Pavel's *Fighter Pull Up Program*.

Again, no "Bondi" chin-ups.

Once you've got those three movements achieved, go and find something else to do with your training. Maybe it is that deadlift or the latest kettlebell challenge. Keep coming back to these three "ups" every now and then, even if it's just to check that you've still got them. These three answer your question: "Am I improving, or maintaining, my independence for tomorrow?"

And there's some space for more deliberate power work with medicine balls, jumps, and whatnot. The key with power is to know your level. An elite athlete's power work is different to someone who's training for tomorrow. You must think of the risk-to-reward ratio. Start looking beyond boring fat loss and focus on building independence instead.

GUIDELINES TO KEEP YOU PROGRESSING

There are a few major, but easy to fix, training mistakes that strike a tuneless chord in my cerebral cortex. If your training and the general feel of your body resembles driving a rusty, Moses-era Swedish Saab, held together by duct tape and chewing gum, the handbrake permanently on, and running on prayers and borrowed time, try the following guidelines.

1. Finish your main meal before dessert

Once you're done with the "main course" of training, do whatever you want to do. It's like eating your steak and broccoli before dominating the chocolate brownie, or polishing off your beans and rice before inhaling the coconut cream and dark chocolate mousse. If you want to do isolated work on your arms, go for it. Pump those suckers up. That's your dessert and you've earned it.

I used to be all "This is the only way to do things and everything else is a waste of time!" I was what you'd call, um, a single-minded jackass. But then I had a Yoda moment: *It's place, everything has.* If that dessert is what makes the training enjoyable for you and keeps you coming back for more, keep doing it. Just eat the potatoes first.

2. Take some time off from training

Once or twice a year put your gym membership on hold for a few weeks, or even a month, and do something else. Keep moving and don't lose the mobility that you've gained through persistent work, but just forget the gym for a little while. Do something else. Go for long bike rides or climb the highest mountain you can find. Hell, play darts and pub trivia, if that's what you enjoy. If you're grinding at the gym 12 months a year, at some point the excitement and fun will fade out. It all becomes, well, a grind. When you allow yourself to have a break, your training will become something to look forward to again.

By the way, this is the rule that I, and some of my advanced clients struggle with the most. But every single time I've taken a step back, my body has thanked me for it. Plan these breaks around holidays to make things convenient.

3. Treat fitness as a tool, not an end goal

I mean, if you are benching 300 kg for reps of 10 and sporting a six-pack 365 days a year, good for you. But if, at the same time, your partner hates your guts and your friends think you're as much fun as watching a Tupperware container rotating in the microwave, you've got to ask yourself what's important. To quote Dan John (once again), who shifted my thinking on training and fitness: "Fitness is an ability to do a task. Nothing else." And that's from a guy who's made a career out of teaching people how to train for better results. His advice is worth listening to.

4. Avoid following the same program for too long

Most of my clients get around six sessions with the same training program before it's time for an update. This doesn't mean we overhaul everything. But we do change a few things around, depending on how they've progressed. This is mostly done by progressing a movement or changing the total intensity and the volume of the program. If the training goals change, there might be a bigger shift on the overall program. The client's training age (how long they've participated in training activities, not just chronological age) plays a part too.

When a program is created specifically for you, it is the best possible program *for you* to follow, *at that time*. But eventually it will be time for you to progress. Done right, your body will adapt to the challenge it is given. The body wants to achieve homeostasis (a fancy word for a stable, fuzzy, warm and comfortable condition, like drinking a hot chocolate in bed while watching *Seinfeld*) and only progresses if it has to. There is only so much you can get out of doing hip bridges on the ground before it's time to advance towards movements that deliver further adaptations. The same goes for the load, reps and sets. Do the same thing over and over and you'll get no further. The definition of insanity, and all.

5. Avoid too much program hopping

This is the opposite of staying with the same program for too long. Most of us know someone who's always looking for the next best thing instead of putting in the work to get the most out of the current program. The coach designing the program has a reason why certain exercises, volumes or loads are done in a certain phase. This is to build you from the ground up. We want to strengthen what's weak, and mobilise and stabilise what's tight, within reason.

When you jump from program to program you reset the clock and never achieve what the program was meant to do. James Clear has a great article on his website JamesClear.com about "staying on the bus" and I highly recommend you read it – it not only applies to training, but also to life and work in general.

6. Stop trying to progress at every session

In a perfect training world, being able to pick up a heavier kettlebell every time you do a goblet squat would be the Holy Grail. In the real world, it doesn't work like that. When you first start out, your progress can be amazing from session to session since the body has so much unused capacity to draw on. Just improving a technique or increasing the range and control of one joint can make you stronger. But even then, progressing every single session isn't always the case. Once your training age increases, the progress feels as slow as waiting for a bus in a once-in-a-decade thunderstorm.

Your performance in the gym can be exceptional if you show up to training fresh after a day of rest. But, if you just blew a major presentation and got verbally abused by your boss who has onion breath I'd bet money that your performance will be down. It's not just poor sleep and eating that affect your training, but also your mental state and level of stress. In the end, and I am risking sounding full of new-age bullshit: your body and mind are one.

To reinforce my message, here's a quote from Buddy Morris, strength and conditioning coach for the Arizona Cardinals:

Your program is a living, breathing organism. It has to adapt to every different circumstance and environment.

Sure, he works with high-level athletes, but don't let that fool you. You have the everyday stress of life, family, your sick pet parrot and a boss with onion breath. That adds up, and usually means that you'll have to be even more accommodating to the fluctuations of life compared to the professional athlete who can focus on training and recovery 24/7.

If your readiness for the day means that you need to halve all the weights and focus on going through the movements with ease, so be it. In the long-term scheme of things, this is the best thing to do. In contrast, if you come in for a low-level movement and mobility session but feel like John Rambo smelling first blood, or Buffy Summers ready to slay the vampire, by all means, get after the weights. This autoregulation becomes easier as your training age increases and you learn to listen to your body better.

THE NEXT FITNESS TREND WON'T SOLVE ALL YOUR PROBLEMS

Every few years (or months, or weeks, depending on who you follow) a new fitness trend sweeps the nation. One thing they all have in common is the promise to give you a better body, or better health and fitness, than you ever thought possible. Many of these are endorsed by celebrities.

Relying on celebrities for health advice makes as much sense as wearing steel-capped thongs on a construction site. Let's ignore what the trainers, clinicians, doctors, researchers and other professionals are saying so we can jump on the next Shake Weight bandwagon. But where there is money to be made, there are always a few twisted (or plain poor informed) souls ready to take advantage over people who are struggling with their health. Or maybe the Shake Weight creators genuinely think that they can help.

But before you throw the baby out with the bathwater, it's not all negative. Some of these past trends are worth keeping in your training arsenal: kettlebells and Indian clubs come to mind. CrossFit may have a bad reputation, but it has gotten more people away from machine training and onto the floor than most of the other "cults" combined. And as much as I don't agree with the religiousness and dogma of the Paleo diet, the shift from processed foods to more vegetables and wholefoods has been great.

When a new trend comes in tomorrow, and it is bound to happen, ask yourself a few questions before buying a ticket and taking the ride: Will this new trend improve my training, fitness and health? Or will it take me away from what is important? Will it add more to my already full and well-balanced plate? Or is it just a fad that's hyped by someone's dad's tanned bodybuilder friend who used to be jacked out of his mind in the mid-80s.

It is unlikely that any new trend is about to emerge that justifies discarding the majority of what you are currently doing. It's more likely that a new trend can change 5% of what you do. At most. Even if it's just to keep you excited about training. That we can accept, as long as it does not do any harm. I've learned to let other people jump in first and if that new thing is still around after a while, I'll give it ago ... provided it looks somewhat sane and doesn't have anything to do with Gwyneth Paltrow.

The big picture

We need to keep our eyes on the big picture: what are you training for? If you are training for tomorrow instead of a competition, there are other and safer ways to get what you are after. Physical therapist and strength coach Charlie Weingroff wrote an excellent article on his website about "lower system loads". He explains how it's possible to create the same amount of force, using lighter loads. He's way smart. But the best thing about the article is that Charlie is a powerlifter at heart, yet he's not all about the big three lifts of squat, bench and deadlift. If you can get the same physical benefits by doing double kettlebell front squats, trapbar deadlifts, swings, single-leg training and other things that don't take as much toll on your body, why wouldn't you? If you can get to the same destination in the same time, while using a safer road, why the hell wouldn't you take it?

So if you run but hate running, and don't plan on competing in it, why do it? Why put your body through the beating that joints take over the period of a long-term running career? Why not use the bike, ropes, or prowler to get the same benefits with less risk? If you hate fishing, why would you get up at 3 am to sit in a boat when you can afford to buy the salmon from the supermarket? It's about getting to the end goal the easiest possible way.

Throughout your training life, keep asking yourself *why* you're doing what you're doing. Know when to stay with the things that work, but also know when to evolve. That way, you are always doing what is best for your body and your goals. Listen to the people who know what they are talking about but also know to differentiate their goals, bodies and minds from your own.

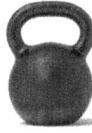

PART 7

The Training Plan For A Resilient Body

This is a semi-customisable and progressive resistance training plan consisting of 24 sessions. By the end of it you'll be stronger, fitter and move better. And if you've implemented the food habits in the book you can also expect to look fitter too, whatever that means these days. But most importantly, you'll have the resilience for the curveballs that life throws at your way.

The resistance program is optimised for twice-a-week training, but it will deliver whether you are doing it once, twice or even three times a week. However, you can expect superior results with twice a week compared to once. Is three better than two then? It depends. Start with two if you can and go from there.

Have a look at the program outline and exercise selection first. Then head over to **RepsAndTheRest.com/SpandexNotCompulsory** to view the exercise demonstrations, and download a program template to fill in the movements that fit you the best. You can also find the templates in Appendix 2 of this book.

If you are at loss about how to perform the exercises (and have watched the instruction videos), depending on your location I might be able to recommend a coach for you to see.

RESET AND MOVEMENT PREPARATION

Each training session starts with Reset and Movement Preparation. The purpose of these movements is to get your body primed for the resistance training part of the program. The Reset and Movement exercises are crucial for your progress, allowing you to make the best and safest possible progress with the program.

Reset and Movement Preparation Exercises

To view demonstration for each exercise, go to
RepsAndTheRest.com/SpandexNotCompulsory

9090 Breathing with a hip lift
Quadruped Breathing
Scapula/Shoulder/Hip CARS
Tactical Frog
Downward Dog to Step to Rotation
Glute Hip Lift
Squat to Stand
Standing Cross Crawl
Farmer Carry (Day A), Suitcase Carry (Day B)

RESILIENCY BUILDING RESISTANCE EXERCISES

Here is where you start to build strength and resiliency through a progressive training plan. You have a list of exercises to choose from depending on your current skill level, experience and how your body feels with certain movements. Here is how your training program looks before you've plugged in your exercises.

Phase 1, Session A		Day 1	Day 2	Day 3	Day 4
Resistance Exercises		weight x reps x sets	weight x reps x sets	weight x reps x sets	weight x reps x sets
A1	Main Lower Body Exercise	x8x2	x8x3	x10x2	x10x3
A2	Main Upper Body Exercise	x8x2	x8x3	x10x2	x10x3
B1	Complementing Lower Body Exercise	x8x2	x8x3	x10x2	x10x3
B2	Complementing Upper Body Exercise	x8x2	x8x3	x10x2	x10x3
B3	Core	3-4 breaths x2	3-4 breaths x3	4-5 breaths x2	4-5 breaths x3

Phase 1, Session B		Day 1	Day 2	Day 3	Day 4
Resistance Exercises		weight x reps x sets	weight x reps x sets	weight x reps x sets	weight x reps x sets
A1	Main Lower Body Exercise	x8x2	x8x3	x10x2	x10x3
A2	Main Upper Body Exercise	x8x2	x8x3	x10x2	x10x3
B1	Complementing Lower Body Exercise	x8x2	x8x3	x10x2	x10x3
B2	Complementing Upper Body Exercise	x8x2	x8x3	x10x2	x10x3
B3	Core	3-4 breaths x2	3-4 breaths x3	4-5 breaths x2	4-5 breaths x3

PHASE 1 – RESILIENCY BUILDING RESISTANCE EXERCISES

PHASE 1, DAY A

A1 Main Lower Body Exercise – choose one

Trapbar Deadlift

Kettlebell Deadlift – often easier to get into the starting position

Romanian Deadlift (off blocks for reduced range of motion, if necessary)

A2 Main Upper Body Exercise – choose one

Push-Ups – see *Focus on Movement Goals to Improve How You Look* for progressions

Dumbbell Bench Press

Dumbbell Floor Press

Complementing Exercises – choose one from each list

B1

Reverse Lunge

Split Squat

Rear Foot Elevated Split Squat

B2

TRX Row

½ Kneeling Cable Row

Chin-Up – see *Focus on Movement Goals to Improve How You Look* for progressions

B3

Supine Overhead Reach

Plank

TRX Fallout

PHASE 1, DAY B

A1 Main Lower Body Exercise – choose one
Goblet Squat

Squat with Reach – easier

Kettlebell Front Squat – harder

A2 Main Upper Body Exercise – choose one
½ Kneeling Landmine Press

½ Kneeling Bottom Up Press

½ Kneeling Single Arm Press

Complementing Exercises – choose one from each list

B1
Single Leg Deadlift

Elevate Squat to Heel Touch

Skater Squat

B2
Split Stance Cable Single Arm Row

Single Arm Dumbbell Row

Renegade Row

B3
Bird Dog

Plank to Arm Slide

TRX Anti-Rotation Pulse

PHASE 2 – RESILIENCY BUILDING RESISTANCE EXERCISES

PHASE 2, DAY A

A1 Power Exercise – choose one
Med Ball Slam
Med Ball Split Stance Slam
Med Ball Single Leg Slam

A2 Core Exercise – choose one
Plank
Supine Overhead Reach
TRX Fallout

B1 Main Lower Body Exercise – choose one
Trapbar Deadlift
Kettlebell Deadlift – often easier to get into the starting position
Romanian Deadlift (off blocks for reduced range of motion, if necessary)

B2 Main Upper Body Exercise – choose one
Push-Ups – see *Focus on Movement Goals to Improve How You Look* for
progressions
Dumbbell Bench Press
Dumbbell Floor Press

Complementing Exercises – choose one from each list

C1
Reverse Lunge
Split Squat
Rear Foot Elevated Split Squat

C2

TRX Row

½ Kneeling Cable Row

Chin-Up – see *Focus on Movement Goals to Improve How You Look* for progressions

PHASE 2, DAY B

A1 Power Exercise – choose one

Med Ball Figure 8 Slam

Med Ball Rotation to Slam

Med Ball Figure 8 Rotation Slam

A2 Core Exercise – choose one

Bird Dog

Plank to Arm Slide

TRX Anti-Rotation Press

B1 Main Lower Body Exercise – choose one

Goblet Squat

Squat with Reach – easier

Kettlebell Front Squat – harder

B2 Main Upper Body Exercise – choose one

½ Kneeling Landmine Press

½ Kneeling Bottom Up Press

½ Kneeling Single Arm Press

Complementing Exercises – choose one from each list

C1

Single Leg Deadlift

Elevated Squat to Heel Touch

Skater Squat

C2

Split Stance Cable Single Arm Row

Dumbbell Row

Renegade Row

PHASE 3 – RESILIENCY BUILDING RESISTANCE EXERCISES

PHASE 3, DAY A

A1 Power Exercise – choose one

Med Ball Rotation to Slam

Med Ball Step to Slam

Med Ball Lateral Step to Slam

A2 Core Exercise – choose one

Plank

Supine Overhead Reach

TRX Fallout

B1 Main Lower Body Exercise – choose one

Trapbar Deadlift

Kettlebell Deadlift – often easier to get into the starting position

Romanian Deadlift (off blocks for reduced range of motion, if necessary)

B2 Main Upper Body Exercise – choose one

Push-Ups – see *Focus on Movement Goals to Improve How You Look* for progressions

Dumbbell Bench Press

Dumbbell Floor Press

Complementing Exercises – choose one from each list

C1
Reverse Lunge
Split Squat
Rear Foot Elevated Split Squat

C2
TRX Row
½ Kneeling Cable Row
Chin-Up – see *Focus on Movement Goals to Improve How You Look* for progressions

PHASE 3, DAY B

A1 Plyometric Exercise – choose one
Skipping Rope (10-30 seconds per set)
Box Jump and Stick
Forward Jump and Stick

A2 Core Exercise – choose one
Bird Dog
Plank to Arm Slide
TRX Anti-Rotation Press

B1 Main Lower Body Exercise – choose one
Goblet Squat
Squat with Reach – easier
Kettlebell Front Squat – harder

B2 Main Upper Body Exercise – choose one
½ Kneeling Landmine Press
½ Kneeling Bottom Up Press
½ Kneeling Single Arm Press

Complementing Exercises – choose one from each list

C1
Single Leg Deadlift

Elevated Squat to Heel Touch

Skater Squat

C2
Split Stance Cable Single Arm Row

Dumbbell Row

Renegade Row

Here is how Phase 1 looks once exercises are filled in, and each session is completed four times:

Phase 1, Session A		Day 1	Day 2	Day 3	Day 4
		Mon 8.1.	Tue 16.1.	Mon 22.1	Tue 30.1
Resistance Exercises		weight x reps x sets	weight x reps x sets	weight x reps x sets	weight x reps x sets
A1	Trapbar Deadlift	75kg x8x2	75kgx8x3	75kg x10x2	75kg x10x3
A2	Push Ups	x8, 7	x8, 8	x9, 7	x10, 7
B1	Reverse Lunge	20kg x8x2	20kg x8x3	20kg x10x2	20kg x10x3
B2	1/2 Kneeling Cable Row	25kg x8x2	25kg x8x3	25kg x10x2	25kg x10x3
B3	Supine Overhead Reach	3-4 breaths x2	3-4 breaths x3	4-5 breaths x2	4-5 breaths x3

Phase 1, Session B		Day 1	Day 2	Day 3	Day 4
		Thu 11.1.	Fri 19.1.	Thu 25.1	Fri 2.2
Resistance Exercises		weight x reps x sets	weight x reps x sets	weight x reps x sets	weight x reps x sets
A1	Goblet Squat	16kg x8x2	16kg x8x3	16x10x2	16kg x10x3
A2	Landmine Press	bar only 20kg x8x2	bar only 20kg x8x3 - easy	22.5kg x10x2	22.5kg x10x3
B1	Single Leg Deadlift	16kg x8x2	16kg x8x3 - easy	20kg x10x2	20kg x10x3
B2	Dumbbell Row	16kg x8x2	16kg x8x3	16kg x10x2	16kg x10x3
B3	Bird Dog	3-4 breaths x2	3-4 breaths x3	4-5 breaths x2	4-5 breaths x3

GENERAL GUIDELINES AND 'HOW TO'

A1, A2

Exercises with the same letter are done as a "circuit". Do all the sets for the given letter i.e. Set 1 of given reps for A1 → Set 1 of given reps for A2 → Set 2 of given reps for A1 → Set 2 of given reps for A2. Once done with all the set, move to B's.

Repetition (Reps)

One complete movement of an exercise. Perform each repetition with a controlled movement.

When the exercise requires counting breaths aim for a 4-second inhale through the nose followed by a powerful 6-second exhale through pursed lips. You can imagine pushing toxic air out of your lungs, get it all out. Try to hold for 2 seconds before inhaling again. That's one rep. It might feel uncomfortable but shouldn't feel like you are suffocating. When inhaling try to get your torso expanding 360 degrees. Not just the stomach or chest.

The speed of each repetition

As a general rule, aim for a 1-second lifting part and 2–3 seconds to get back to the starting position. You are in control, not the weight or the gravity. (Also, fight the gravity. How's that for a challenge?)

Set

A group of consecutive reps performed without rest.

Choosing the ideal weight

If the goal is to complete eight repetitions for three sets find a weight that allows no more than 10 repetitions on the first set. If you can do 12, the weight is too light. If you can only do six, the weight is too heavy.

As you get stronger and have a better idea of your weights you can use the Delorme Method:

1st set – choose a weight that is 50% of what you can do for the given rep range (i.e. if you can do eight reps with 100 kg, use 50 kg).

2nd set – choose a weight that is 75% of what you can for the given rep range (i.e. if you can do eight reps with 100 kg, use 75 kg).

3rd set – choose a weight that is 100% of what you can for the given rep range (i.e. if you can do eight reps with 100 kg, use 100 kg).

When the increments between weights are too big

With kettlebells or dumbbells the increases between weights are often in 4 kg. It is common that a Goblet Squat is somewhat easy with 20 kg but too challenging at 24 kg. This is how you can still progress:

If you can do all the sets and repetitions (i.e. eight repetitions for three sets) with a 20 kg kettlebell:

1. slow down the movement, add a few second pause at the bottom, or

2. add a repetition to each set, or

3. use a 24 kg kettlebell and do as many repetitions as you can without losing form. It might look like this:

- 1st set: 8 reps

- 2nd set: 6 reps

- 3rd set: 5 reps

Rest between sets / exercises

As a general rule aim for somewhere around 60–120 seconds before moving from an exercise to another. If it takes you more than 2 minutes to recover there is a chance that the weight is too heavy. If you are ready to go with less than 45 seconds of rest, the weight is probably not heavy enough. These are not cardio sessions, you want the extra rest so that each set is perfect, and you get the most out of your strength sessions.

Single leg and single arm exercises

The given rep ranges are always per side, i.e. "Rear Foot Elevated Split Squat 8 reps for 3 sets" means do eight reps with your left leg, followed by eight reps on your right leg. That's one set.

When something hurts

A bit of discomfort and muscle soreness is OK and expected. But if it's beyond the usual feeling that you get from exercising a muscle, or if you feel like it's joint or nerve pain, please stop. Either seek coaching to confirm you are performing each exercise correctly or see a physical therapist or another clinician to get to the source of your pain. "No pain, no gain" is an idiotic term and doesn't lead to a resilient body.

CONDITIONING OPTIONS

If you are just getting started

Easy, long steady-state conditioning – aim for 60 minutes once or twice a week. Keep a pace where you can comfortably keep a conversation going. Treadmill, cross trainer, cycling, hiking all work fine. Even swimming if you're good at it. Being outdoors is dope.

If you have been doing long, steady-state conditioning for at least four weeks

Moderate conditioning – aim for once or twice a week, while still doing the long, steady-state conditioning. Treadmill, cross trainer, cycling all work fine. Being outdoors is still dope. Keep a pace for 30 minutes where you can barely keep a conversation going.

Or try rucking. Load up a backpack with 10–20 kilograms of weight and go for a 30-minute walk. A great idea I got from an article by Tim Anderson of *Original Strength.*

If you have been doing moderate conditioning for at least four weeks

Moderate to hard conditioning – aim for once every week or fortnight, while still doing the long, steady-state conditioning and moderate conditioning. Do a 20–30 second sprint, followed by 40–60 second recovery. Keep the recovery longer than the effort. Repeat anywhere between 2–10 times, depending on your current level of conditioning. You can try any of the following: hill or stair run (avoid if you end up getting knee or any other joint pain), indoor cycling (easy to set up, relatively easy on the joints), swimming (easy on the joints). Being in the water is dope.

If you are 100% confident with a kettlebell swing you could use that too by doing a 10–20 second effort with a 40–50 second rest.

If you are confident with your form with resistance exercises you can also set up a circuit. Try 30 seconds with each exercise, followed by a 60-second rest before moving on to the next one:

⊙ TRX Row

⊙ Goblet Squat

⊙ Push-Ups

⊙ Reverse Lunge

⊙ Farmer Walk

Repeat one to two times. Drop the ego and stay honest to yourself. If you know your form is sloppy stop before the end of the 30-second mark.

Again, muscle discomfort and a higher heart rate (that also recovers quickly) are good for you. But there is no gain in pain in any of this.

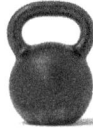

PART 8

Look At All The Food I Can Eat

IF YOU STRUGGLE WITH FAT LOSS

There are no magic tricks or lifestyle hacks to speed up the process of improving how your body feels, looks and functions, and there's only so many books you can read until you have to commit to doing the hard stuff. The work. The change. Achieving fat loss can be as hard as it gets. Not even Dr Oz can help you here, no matter what he might want you to believe.

What you need is common-sense practices, sacrifices and patience. A lot of patience. Fat loss is not meant to be easy. If you don't struggle with your weight, I am sure you know someone who does. It's an epidemic in our convenience-driven society that relies on quick fixes to move from one calorie hit to the next. We live from meal to meal instead of thinking about the long-term consequences. If you are complaining about your struggle with fat loss while being aware of how unhealthy your diet is, you are pondering a mathematically illogical question: you are asking yourself why 1+1=2. Why can't it be 3?

Some things are non-negotiable when it comes to fat loss. One of them is that you can't get there if you are consuming more calories than you burn. Mathematically, it doesn't make sense. If you eat 2,200 calories a day while your body only burns 2,100, at the end of the week you will have accumulated an extra 700 calories. Over a month that equals roughly 2,800 calories. Over a year: 36,400 calories. Once you take into consideration that most of us are more likely to overeat and indulge over the weekends and holidays, the yearly total could be significantly more than what I have estimated above.

One higher-calorie meal here and there does not make a difference to your weight when you are eating healthily 85–90% of the time. But multiple high-calorie days throughout the week will add up without you even noticing. You don't suddenly wake up 10 kg heavier than yesterday. It happens over time and you have the power to stop it.

This brings us back to the point that losing weight is hard. Really hard. You are bombarded with high-calorie (and ridiculously tasty) meals and treats at every turn. Maybe you are so used to eating the saltiest, fattiest and sweetest meals that you can't appreciate the flavours in more basic, healthy, home-cooked meals. Or maybe it is that we, as a society, have lost the ability to make basic, healthy, home-cooked meals tasty.

Our society applauds the skills that advance your career and makes you (or the company) money. In turn, we sacrifice our health for the next promotion. Then we spend that hard-earned cash trying to regain the health we once had. What we should do instead is to champion the skills that keep us healthy. We know everything about the possible fluctuations of the stock market and the functions of all the keyboard shortcuts on our laptops. Yet we don't know how to boil a damn egg. Or, we "don't have time" to boil an egg.

It's not about how busy you are. It's about what you prioritise in life. If you want to cook and eat healthily, if your health is as valuable to you as your career, I am sure you can find time for it. You'll find time by eliminating whatever is unnecessary.

I get it; it's hard. I struggled to write this chapter. I struggled because I chose to do other things with my time. But I'm not sitting in the corner cursing my life because I don't have time. I acknowledge that I spent time on something else and I'm paying for it now by having to set my alarm for 5.30 am on Sunday, and piss off my wife because the alarm wakes her up too. But I digress. If you are tearing your hair out while struggling to shift your weight, it's time to ask yourself two questions:

1. "What is important?"

If the answer to the above question is something other than your health or losing fat, that's cool. Now you've acknowledged it. You can stop feeling anxiety over prioritising other things above your health. You can move on and focus on the things that are important to you right now instead.

However, if you answer that your health is important, it's time to answer the second question:

2. "Am I doing everything that is in my power to get the results that I want?"

If you are, good for you. If not, stop wondering and start doing. Start by changing one thing for the next four weeks. Choose something that will have a positive impact on your health over the long term. Imagine yourself in two years' time: you've successfully dropped your weight and are living a lighter, happier and healthier life. What habits does that person (you in two years, that is) do every day?

Keep in mind that this won't be easy. There will be struggles. But if it's important to you, it's all worth it. And it gets easier over time.

Maybe it all starts by boiling an egg.

YOU CAN'T OUT-TRAIN AN UNHEALTHY DIET

There is no doubt that training more and with higher intensities will give you more flexibility with your diet. It can help you to build a buffer zone for calories so that the extra piece of Aunt Betty's cheesecake is less likely to park itself on your waist. That's all positive. That being said, over-exercising to balance out an unhealthy diet is not the best, nor the safest, way to build a fitter and healthier body that will be able to weather the storms of life.

The negatives of excessive training

Long periods of high-volume and high-intensity training are taxing on your body and can lead to injury, burnout or an impaired immune system. There will also come a time when this frequency of exercise is not possible. It's not sustainable when life is busy. If your training intensity is the only thing that's keeping your weight in check, it's difficult to resort to eating birdseed when you can't train with the usual intensity.

The more sustainable approach is to get on top of your eating habits. This doesn't mean following restrictive diets, but creating habits that allow flexibility during the times that are out of the ordinary.

Flexible, healthier eating habits in real life

Let's stop acting like there's a fine line between "healthy" and "unhealthy". Instead, imagine there is a large area with a lot of room in each direction. Having flexible eating habits makes busy times more manageable compared to just trying to out-train your diet. But it also allows you to move away from training programs that only focus on fat loss.

Let's explore three common groups that people seem to fall into when it comes to eating habits.

1. "I DON'T CARE"

For this group, pretty much anything edible goes. Want to have nachos and Cheerios with chocolate milk and ice-cream for breakfast? They will have at it.

You might be stuck in this section because you think that you have to choose between this and the next group.

2. "I CARE WAY TOO MUCH"

These folks have an extremely narrow view of what a "healthy" diet is. People in this group might freak out if they can't get an accurate number of calories, or the macronutrient split of each meal. It's like trying to balance on top of a triangle: not only is it hard, but also extremely uncomfortable.

Unless you are a professional athlete (even then, this is debatable) or someone with an extremely restrictive health condition, you don't need to be one of these people. Unfortunately, people new to healthy eating often start here. I believe it's also the reason why most people who start get disheartened and stop early.

If you are just moving away from the "I don't care" group, you might think this is the way to go. All or nothing. The hardcore side of the fitness industry says if you're not here, you're not trying hard enough. The dietary zealots chime in with their scare tactics: "Don't eat this or else you'll cause inflammation, obesity, gout and nuclear war".

I used to sit in this group. I thought carbs were evil, something that God created on the eighth day just to pester the mankind. It's not a great place to be for flourishing physical and mental happiness.

3. "I CARE JUST ENOUGH"

In the middle there's the group of people who have a lot of room and flexibility for trial and error. For most people, like you and me, this is where we want to be. Some days ice-cream is on the menu and some days it's not. And it's OK. These people have healthy but flexible eating habits and they build up to two to four days of purposeful training per week. They stay active outside of the training sessions and don't let stress get the better of them. So, does this still work if I'm training for fat loss?

Yes. Focus on strength and movement skills instead acting like the Duracell Bunny high on speed. The best training program for fat loss is still a strength-based, lower-repetition plan. This helps you to maintain or even gain muscle mass when your food plan is lower in calories than usual. If you only do high-repetition, lighter-weight sessions, you might as well just do cardio. The downside of only doing cardio is that it does not preserve the lean muscle mass the same way as heavy strength training does. You will feel exhausted after each session, leaving the gym more tired than when you came in. This combined with lower calories means you will lose weight but a lot of it will be muscle mass.

You'll end up with the typical "skinny-fat" body. Yes, I hate that term too, but that's what happens. Besides that, being on a typical "fat loss training plan" for the long term is boring as batshit. Eventually the hamster wheel will get the better of you.

So, lift heavy, become strong and more independent, increase your bone density and preserve or even build muscle. But if you are trying to out-train an unhealthy diet with excessive fitness endeavours, you are not aligning your actions with your goals. You are climbing the wrong ladder. Reaching for the wrong star. Sealing the wrong window. You get the point. It's like trying to build a massive deadlift by only working on bench presses. Eventually you'll have to pull the bar off the floor too. For fat loss, that means harvesting patience and pouring most of your efforts into building healthier eating habits. Then train because it makes you strong and maintains, or even builds, lean muscle. You'll be "in shape" and look healthy. But you don't necessarily look like Brad Pitt in *Fight Club* or Jessica Alba in *Into the Blue.* And that's cool too.

Fuck "cheat" meals

Why do we label every treat or an out-of-the-ordinary meal as a "cheat" meal? What or who are we cheating? Life? Ourselves? The coaches and trainers we hire?

Food is not "good" or "bad". Food has no feelings or morals. It doesn't believe in a certain god or follow a particular political party. At its core, (and this is me getting deep into science) food sustains life. It keeps us from dying of starvation.

We like to be able to identify "good" and "bad" foods because these labels make diets simple, giving us clear-cut rules to follow instead of thinking for ourselves, tuning into our hunger cues and making decisions about what our body needs at that moment.

Unless you have some life-threatening allergies, or a *real* moral or spiritual dilemma, every single food item has its place in a healthy diet. Sure, some are meant to be had more often than others, such as carrots over fries. But neither of them is "better" or "worse" than the other. In my suburban life I choose carrots more often than fries because I know their nutrition density keep me closer to my goal of being healthy. But if I was shipwrecked on a desert island with no other food sources in sight, give me fries over carrots any day. Fries destroy carrots when it comes to the battle of calories for survival, and that's all I would care about at that point. I couldn't give two shits about vitamins and minerals when I am about to die of hunger. Does that make carrots a bad food? Does it mean that fries are good?

Instead of thinking about food as either morally "good" or bad", think about food as a tool which can bring you closer to your goals, keep you where you are, or move you further away from your goals. What will bring you closer to where you want to be?

When you eat a diet suitable for adults you do not need to worry about when you're allowed a cheat meal. You don't need to count the days until you can eat something delicious again on the weekend. Depending on your situation, lifestyle and goals, only you can make the decision about what you should eat.

Now, all that being said, you still need to build habits from the ground up to get to this point. But they don't have to involve meal plans and labelling "good" and "bad" foods.

BEING HEALTHY WITHOUT HATING LIFE

There are some habits that are crucial for your quest to get healthy (and stay there) while maintaining sanity and balance in life. I guarantee that if you work towards owning these habits (one at a time, of course), you are well on your way to becoming a healthier version of yourself. I haven't included specific macronutrient ratios or total calories because what's right for you is different to your friend Rick or Renata who lives down the street. It depends on your body type, lifestyle and values, just to name a few. And to be honest, advising people on specific macronutrients is beyond my scope of practice. You need to talk to a dietitian to sort that shit out. But often, getting all Stephen Hawking over calories and macros becomes irrelevant once these habits are in place. After all, this is not space-science.

Prioritise protein and vegetables

WHY?

Your body functions better when it gets enough nutrients, vitamins and minerals. Proteins (amino acids) are responsible for our structure, hormone function, enzymes and immune function. As stated in *The Essentials of Sport and Exercise Nutrition Certification Manual* by Precision Nutrition, "While carbohydrate and fat balance is quite well maintained in the body, it's quite difficult to maintain protein balance without adequate protein intake." Eating meals higher in protein will also improve satiety, which in turn can help with unnecessary snacking.

Vitamins and minerals (sourced from vegetables) have several regulatory functions in the body. Deficiencies in these cause poor health, increased disease risk, obesity and more.

HOW?

→ Protein requirements differ wildly depending on sex, body type and activity level. As a minimum, eat at least three palm sizes of protein-rich foods each day.

→ As a minimum, eat at least four fistfuls of vegetables each day. More is better here.

→ Eat a wide range of different vegetables.

→ Think your diet as a bucket: fill the bucket with big rocks (these rocks are your vegetables and protein). Then pour sand in the bucket to fill in the gaps (this sand is everything else that you might want/ need to eat: for some it's a lot of carbohydrates, for others it's more fat, and for some it's both). Don't build your diet around processed foods that are often lower in protein and nutrients.

→ If you think you are low in certain vitamins or minerals I recommend getting your levels checked by a health professional who is well-versed in nutrient deficiencies.

Enter sandman

WHY?

You can't keep raging around like a mad bear. Even the maddest bear chills out every now and then and sits down to eat some forest berries. Additionally, even the maddest bear sleeps throughout the winter. Your body needs deep sleep to repair itself. Your strength doesn't actually improve during your workouts; it improves while recovering optimally from training.

If you are constantly sleep-deprived, you're probably making less-than-ideal decisions about your health, work and family, which can result in suboptimal physical and mental health. If you think that you're wasting time sleeping because it cuts your days shorter, I've got news for you: walking zombies are not efficient. You will get more done in a shorter time when you are well rested. You will also have smaller bags under your eyes, which in itself is dope to see in the mirror.

If none of that makes you a sleep enthusiast, I hope this will: lack of sleep negatively affects your fat-loss efforts.

HOW?

- Again, everyone's different, but I am yet to meet anyone who functions well with less than seven hours of sleep. Try sleeping seven, eight, nine or even more hours a night and see what makes you feel the best.

- Establish a bedtime routine. Follow it every night.

- Manage your stress better.

- Invest in a proper bed and mattress.

Have flexibility in your diet

WHY?

As we've established, eating doesn't always have to be perfect. You won't always have the option to choose a healthy meal. Sometimes you won't even want to. You want to be able to go out with people and break bread with them, have a few drinks and generally let the good times roll. There are more important things to do than constantly worry about how each food will affect your body.

In our quest for simplifying a complex topic, we are drawn towards meal plans, like they are the Holy Grail of sustainable body transformation. Meal plans work, until they don't. Imagine your meal plan required you to prep your week's worth of food on Sunday afternoon, and then a friend calls in an emergency. Or you're called in to work at the last minute. Or you come down with the flu. The meal prep doesn't get done. When something happens in life that forces us off the perfect, balanced, well-oiled rails, we have no idea what to do because all we ever did was follow rules instead of learning principles and working on skills to use when life is not perfect. And we all know that life is not perfect.

HOW?

- For 80–90% of the time, stick with nutrient-rich wholefoods that make your body feel good. You know this: vegetables, meat, fish, legumes, nuts, starchy vegetables, fruit.

- Eat mostly meals that are cooked from fresh, unprocessed ingredients.

- When going out or eating something that's not considered a wholefood, don't feel guilty or think you have to earn your food through extra training. But don't binge either. Eat the same way as you would eat any other meal: slow and mindfully.

- As long as you are moving in the right direction with your health or staying where you want to stay, you are doing it right, for you. Slow progress that lasts is better than a strict, quick fix that fades.

Learn how to cook

WHY?

This might be the most important skill to have for leading a healthy life. If you don't know how to cook it's harder to be proactive about your food choices. You will be restricted to what is available around you, or what others feel like cooking for you. Even if you eat out most of the time, knowing what ingredients go in different dishes will help you to navigate the healthier options.

Besides, your partner, family and friends will love the fact that you can whip up a delicious, healthy meal in no time.

HOW?

- Learn the basic skills of chopping, frying, braising, steaming, and boiling. You don't have to master them; just knowing *how* to do them is enough to start.

- Understand the basics of flavour matching. Know what goes well with different ingredients. This might be one of the most important skills when it comes to cooking. Just knowing how to make a simple salad dressing or stir-fry sauce will get you far. Hint number one: less is more. Hint number two: when in doubt, add salt and pepper. Hint number three: Cajun spice goes with everything.

- Keep your kitchen stocked with basic ingredients. There's nothing worse than getting home and realising that all you have in the fridge is a jar of pickled onions, half a carton of week-old milk and a can of white paint for the outdoor deck.

Listen to hunger cues

WHY?

It's harder to overeat if you only eat when you are actually hungry. It's better for your long-term sanity to be aware of your hunger cues and feelings of fullness than it is to keep adding up calories in an app throughout the day. Eating is meant to be a pleasant experience, not an exercise in maths.

When eating slowly, every bite you take is a Riverdance on your tastebuds. You'll get more out of each forkful. When eating treats this way, you are more aware of the flavours and become satisfied with less. You are more likely to get the satiated feeling that "I've had enough", compared to rushing through a bowl of ice-cream in 2 minutes flat (including licking the bowl) without really noticing the taste at all.

It also takes a while for your stomach to send the signals of fullness to your brain. If you rush through your meal of meatballs you are more likely to end up feeling stuffed. That in turn will make you lethargic and possibly give you indigestion.

HOW?

⊘ Acknowledge hunger for 60 minutes (or less, if too challenging) before eating to be sure that you are actually hungry and not just bored and looking for something to do, or confusing the feeling of thirst with the feeling of hunger. I got this idea from Georgie Fear's *Lean Habits* book and it's been a gamechanger for myself and a bunch of my clients.

⊘ Eat without rushing. Take at least 20 bites with each forkful, placing the fork on the table between each mouthful. This is almost an unbearable challenge for most.

- Be mindful and fully present. If watching TV or scrolling Facebook makes you less mindful, turn it off.

- Stop eating when you feel "just right". Vague? Maybe, but if you practise, you'll get to know how this feels.

- I recommend you pick up a copy of Georgie Fear's *Lean Habits* book.

Eat according to your activity levels and body type

WHY?

If you spend eight hours a day sitting at your desk, your calorie requirements will be vastly different to someone who works in a mine shovelling dirt for eight hours a day. If your choice of sport is darts, your fuelling tactics should be different to someone who lifts weights for an hour each day.

HOW?

- Keep your protein and vegetable serves the same but play around with your carbohydrate and fat intake. See if you feel better and get the desired results with higher carbohydrates and a lower fat intake, or if you are better off with lower carbohydrates and a higher fat intake.

- If you are feeling tired and lethargic, increase your carbohydrates first and see how you react. If you are feeling better and getting the results you want, keep doing it. If not, change something and reassess.

Manage stress

WHY?

Stress causes hormonal imbalances in your body that affect your fat-burning capabilities as well as overall health. We make worse decisions when under stress. Stress also affects your sleep, and lack of sleep is the evil enemy of health.

HOW?

- Meditate

- Learn to play. Do something fun that is not considered productive. Paint, dance, draw, write, play curling, head bang to a Machine Head song or shred your air guitar to "Rocket queen".

- Live in the now. Read the first half of *The Power of Now* by Eckhart Tolle (personally, the second half is barely good enough for lighting a fireplace).

- Keep a gratitude journal. Life seems good once you start adding up the little things. Too often we let them pass without fully appreciating them.

Raise less hell with your drinking

WHY?

I think this is obvious but it's too important not to mention. Big drinking sessions not only add a huge spike to your calorie intake but also affect your overall health. You are more likely to make poorer eating decisions when hitting the cans. The effects of a hangover carry well over to the next week. It'll affect your training sessions as well as your mental capacity to get stuff done. It's also an idiotic way to release stress.

I am not saying that I am a saint of the alcohol-free universe. I, too, have a few too many now and then, but it's few and far between. I hate how it makes me feel the next day(s).

HOW?

- If you are having trouble stopping, ask yourself if there is a void you are trying to fill.

- Could you replace the drinking with another, more productive, activity?

- Is it always certain people that you raise hell with? Damn you, Hank Moody. Hang out with other people.

- Enjoy a drink or five but don't get drunk every weekend. I honestly don't know what else to say here.

- Still struggling? It might be worth getting some help with your drinking.

DECISION POINTS TO IMPROVE EATING HABITS

In his book *Two Awesome Hours*, Josh Davis draws from his experience in neuroscience to write about how to be effective with our work instead of solely focusing on efficiency.

One of the biggest themes of his book is to learn to take advantage of what he calls "decision points". These are the moments when we snap out of our workflow before tackling another item on our to-do list. The usual way is to jump into the next task straight away. But he argues that we should savour these moments and use them to decide what's important instead of what's urgent – a principle also used by Stephen R Covey in *The 7 Habits of Highly Effective People*, and explored earlier in this book. It might even mean letting our minds wander for a short time before coming back to the present.

We should use similar decision points to our advantage to improve our eating habits. I guess, in a way, it all comes back to mindfulness. Most of the time we function on autopilot; our actions are non-conscious routines. It doesn't mean that we are not aware of our actions, but, rather, that they are well-rehearsed and learned and require only a little conscious monitoring. Think about brushing your teeth or changing gears in a car. Most of the time it's good that we go on autopilot as it saves us a lot of decision-making, therefore saving mental energy for difficult and important tasks. The problem is that we use these same automated habits to make less than optimal choices with our eating. We wolf our way through a bowl of M&M's, a fistful at a time, while tackling the curveballs that our job throws our way. We do it on autopilot.

What if instead, when you feel the urge to eat, whether out of boredom or actual hunger, you take a moment, look away from the computer or take a short stroll and ask yourself what you really feel like. What would make you feel better for the rest of the day? Do you need a small or large serve? Savoury or sweet? Crisp or soft? Are you hungry in the first place? Once you listen to what you want, you are more likely to eat a moderate amount of it until you are satisfied instead of mindlessly consuming everything in sight. It's all about attention and intention. Of course, if you've planned ahead and prepared or ordered a healthy meal, this decision is easy. If you indeed are hungry.

And once you have the meal in front of you, take your time while eating. Don't try to work at the same time; don't check Facebook or email. Just eat. Instead of shoving food in like it has legs, stop briefly after each mouthful to check in: am I getting full, have I had enough? What flavours can I taste? Does this cracker taste like cardboard? Would I enjoy this banana more after peeling it? Not only will you have more energy after the meal as you don't end up overeating, you will also taste all the flavours in the food, making the whole experience more enjoyable.

For the love of a donut

One of my extremely busy clients was able to implement some of these decision points with his donut-eating habit. He absolutely loves donuts (then again, who doesn't?). He explained how he had been able to curb his donut consumption by simply asking himself the question "Is this reward worth the consequences?" He is not asking the question to guilt himself out of eating the donut, but rather to question if the brief moment of passion shared with the donut brings enough pleasure to justify the post-donut effects.

He went on to explain that even if he cuts the donut into small pieces and eats it slowly, it will only take him 1 or 2 minutes to eat it. So he thought to himself, are those few minutes worth the sluggish feeling he has to deal with afterwards?

Lately, he has come think of the sweet taste from another perspective because of what it reminds him of. He has associated the sweet taste with the fact that it will make him feel sluggish. He still loves the taste of sugar, but not what it does to him, which makes him question this whole situation involving donuts. I am blown away by the simplicity of the whole thing.

There is nothing wrong with eating donuts, but if it's gone in 60 seconds without any further enjoyment, with a few hours of negative effects, is it really worth it?

HEALTHY EATING IS NOT A BANDWAGON FROM WHICH YOU FALL

Healthy eating doesn't have to be about repeatedly jumping on and falling off a bandwagon, it's more like a self-powered vehicle. Like a bicycle. It's completely up to us to pedal away, sometimes gaining momentum, sometimes slowing down to take the scenic route. There will be bumps in the road and flat tyres, but we keep fixing ourselves up and pedaling one revolution after the other. No matter how slow or steady, we will eventually end up in front of those who've steamed ahead on the bandwagon and then come crashing off. After all, there are birthday parties to attend, popcorn at the movies, times when you sit on the couch and tune into your favourite TV show with a bowl of chocolate-chip ice-cream. Then there are office Christmas parties with way too much alcohol lying around – that devil's elixir ruining all your hard work in the gym and asking you to commit unthinkable things, all in the name of baby Jesus.

Do these holiday-season clickbait headlines sound familiar? "How to beat the Christmas calorie explosion." "How to navigate the temptations of holiday eating." "Five ways to say 'no' to your mum's casserole so you can still see your bicep veins on January 1st". And my personal favourite: "Ten microwave-friendly Christmas recipes using only organic chicken, free-range egg whites and holy broccoli (number 7 will surprise you)."

OK, so maybe it's not quite that bad. But it's easy to prey on people's insecurities. So instead of buying into this restrictive, guilt-laden propaganda, let me explain my thoughts on the best possible actions you can take when your next party or holiday rolls around.

Learn to let go without being out of control

Learning to let go is hard. If you have been working on your eating and training habits for a while now, you have undoubtedly created some rules for yourself. Maybe you've learned what type of eating works the best for your body. Maybe you've got some amazing results and you are afraid that the holiday is going to reverse all of it. You are afraid you will revert back to your old self.

To know how to let go at the right times and still stay in control is an art form. And the only way to get better at it is to practise and lean into the uncomfortable. If you want to get better at something, there comes a time when you can't rely on the training wheels anymore. You can't rely on someone holding you upright. You'll have to try to balance on your own. You might fall a couple of times in the beginning. And all you can do is learn from it, get back on the bike, master all your determination and have another go.

By "letting go" I mean that it is OK not to be on your A-game all the time. It's OK to eat a fruit-mince pie or two, and not feel like you've failed at life. It's OK to have a fifth beer. It's OK to eat Mum's casserole, even if it has a triple-cheese crust. The key is to be in the moment, enjoy every bite you take and just have some good times without worrying about how many calories this meal or drink has. Again, if your eating and training habits are in place 80–90% of the time, that last 10–20% doesn't make *any* difference in the long run.

I preach mindful eating because it allows you to let go and still be in control. Food is meant to make you feel good and it is meant to be shared with friends and family through important times in life. When you are mindful, you can enjoy special meals and still not overeat.

You don't have to do "damage control"

It's not about how hard you can hit the gym next week and undo all the "damage" that you've done. You don't have to restrict your calories. You don't have to go on a "juice cleanse" (this is bullshit anyway; there's a reason we have this thing called a "liver"). Having the mindset that you have to earn your food by doing more exercise is a doomed plan: all it does is create negative thoughts about training. Training and movement become a punishment instead of something that you should be grateful for being able to do.

No: the very next day is a clean slate. Just go back to your healthy eating habits. And if the next day brings few more mince pies and couple of beers, so be it. Just make a conscious choice about it.

I hope you get the point I am trying to make here. I am not saying you should eat seven cheese casseroles and drink two cases of beer every day for a month. Because it won't make you feel good (unless that's the sort of thing you're into). I am not saying you should throw out all the healthy habits you've worked so hard for. No, sprinkle them into your holiday. Keep the fire burning. They are flexible, remember. They change as you and your circumstances change. Enjoy food and drinks mindfully and guilt-free, and have good times with the people that you care about. If you can't get to the gym for a month due to various reasons, it's OK. There are a million other things you can do and still stay active. And none of them have to feel like exercise.

Allowing yourself to have a break doesn't mean that you've failed in humanity. Being mindful about your choices and being in the moment means that you don't have to restart each time.

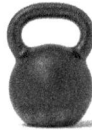

PART 9

Calm And Grace = Health

ATTITUDE FOR HAPPINESS

Most of us have big aspirations for the future. If you're like me, you're always looking for the next thing to work on or to get better at. Maybe you want to learn a new language, build a better body or master the trumpet. There's a force pushing you, so you tend to jump onto another project as soon as the previous task is done. You don't want to waste a single day of your life feeling as if you didn't accomplish something meaningful. If you are anything like me, you might have a tendency to seek happiness in perfection. But I think we're doing it wrong. Happiness can be found by simply shifting our attitude.

Do you take time to stop and think about what you've accomplished after each project and after each win? Do you take a moment to appreciate what you have created, learned, or how you have bettered yourself? Maybe you just switched from eating takeaway seven days a week to only on the weekends. It might seem small, but did you consider the scale of improvement that it has for your long-term health (and your wallet)?

Or, like me, did you move on without sparing a second thought for what you accomplished?

A while back I was on one of my regular long walks and I had an epiphany. Something just clicked. Even though I'd heard and read this from a dozen or more sources over the past few years, I never truly *got it* until that moment. This time, I felt it on a deeper level than ever before. I realised that I only have *now*. I realised that if I always look to the future and work towards a new thing, that "perfect future", I will miss most things happening *today*. I always thought that I had been living in the present, yet I hadn't. At all.

Living for *now* doesn't mean that you shouldn't learn new things, improve your body or have something to look forward to in your trumpet classes. You absolutely should! But you shouldn't allow yourself to believe that the one thing you are chasing is the one magical addition your life is missing. If you forget to be present as life happens today, nothing will change as you get older. You will always use all your energy working towards something better, but you will keep moving the goalposts each time.

Remind yourself about something that you worked extremely hard to achieve, and were finally able to make a reality. Was the feeling in the end as glorious as you thought it would be? Did that feeling last?

Actions for finding contentment

There are a few things that I do every day that help me to be more content.

For one, I try to appreciate seemingly unimportant everyday moments that come my way. I will try to look for the upside in even the seemingly negative things. When something doesn't work out the way I wanted, I try not to blame myself or look for others to blame. I try to objectively observe the situation to find ways to do better next time. This puts me in the driver's seat.

When I am looking forward to something in the near future, I try not to let it consume all of my thinking. Otherwise I miss all the days leading up to it, and often the planning and the excitement that comes with it is half the fun.

When I hear a song that moves me, I stop and take it all in. I appreciate that someone put in the work to make an amazing piece of music. I feel grateful that I can hear the sound funneling through the pinna into the auditory canal.

Each time I get home, one of our cats, in a very un-catlike way, sprints to the door to greet me. It's weird, cute and awesome all at the same time. And no matter how tired, hungry or irritable I might feel, I take a minute or two to pat him. Because one day he won't be there.

What little moments can you appreciate in your everyday life? What things make you feel content? Is it being the best parent, daughter, brother, partner you can be? Maybe it's doing charity work or achieving a certain status or position in your professional life.

Eliminate the negatives where possible

I've also been ruthless about cutting out stuff that doesn't make me happy. I only hang out with people whose company I enjoy, and I do what I can to eliminate tasks that I irritate me. Yes, I still vacuum and do the dishes. But hey, a clean house makes the wife happy.

Is there room in your life to cut out what doesn't make you happy? Think about what adjustments you can make to get a little closer to that perfect day. Don't make your decisions based on what others might think of you. Some of the decisions required are tough, awkward, inconvenient and go against the current of what everyone else thinks you should do. But if you are following what feels right for you, it will make you more content. In essence: care more about what you care about and care less about what other people think.

How about fitness goals?

With fitness goals, it's easy to fall into the trap of constantly moving the goalposts. To avoid this, it's important to see contentment as the goal instead of an ideal weight or body type. Work to improve your health, body composition or strength, but find gratitude in what you have at this moment. Even if you are not 100% satisfied with how you currently look or feel (who is, anyway?), remind yourself of what is awesome about your body today.

There is one thing in life that you can't get back or make more of, and that is time. Focus on the process and consistency of doing the right things for you and eventually you will get where you want to go to. You might as well enjoy the ride. And each time you take a positive action, embrace it as if you've won. Because you did.

THE SKILL OF BEING STILL

The other day, I was sitting on the bus on the way home minding my own business as I usually do. Yet I was drawn to observe the erratic behaviour of the gentleman sitting in front of me. A gentleman who we shall call Homer. It looked as if Homer's mind and fingers were possessed by mystic, dark forces. Something out of a zombie apocalypse. He couldn't stop tapping and swiping at his phone. Nothing new there. Sometimes you need to get work done and in a pinch a smartphone can act as a vehicle for productivity. I get that. But he wasn't being productive. Rather, he followed the cycle of:

check email – check messages – check email – use the calculator – check messages – check Facebook – check Whatsapp – check the news – check email – do another round of calculation – go back to beginning and repeat it all.

He wasn't doing thorough research on something that he needed urgent information about. No, it was a quick 2–3 seconds in each app before moving on to the next. On a few occasions he opened the app, closed it immediately and repeated the same for two or three apps before settling on one app for a maximum of 5 seconds. It wasn't as if he was receiving any messages or emails, yet he was on a constant lookout for them. It was amusing, sad and exhausing to watch it unfolding. He was constantly seeking something, and was oblivious that he was stuck in this unrewarding loop.

This has become our norm

Being still and *not* doing anything is hard. That's why we resort to smartphone slavery, nail-biting (guilty!), smoking or social drinking. These activities calm us down when we feel uncomfortable. They make us look busy and distract our mind from the fact that we are uncomfortable being with ourselves. You doubt this? Next time you are waiting for your morning latte, look around you. How many people can you see doing nothing? None. They're likely to be distracting themselves with phones, tablets, laptops, e-readers and whatnot. Here's a challenge my friend Bec once asked me to do: See how long you can stand still with your arms hanging relaxed on each side. Don't check your phone or cross your arms. Just stand. It's uncomfortable.

Why should you care?

Because life is better when you are comfortable with yourself. If you always distract yourself by being surrounded with minor busyness, activities, or other people because you are not comfortable with who you are, how can you expect to ever find contentment with what you've got? The other people or busyness stop you from reflecting on what is going on with *you*. Some of us live without ever being comfortable in our own company.

I believe that happiness and contentment begin by first knowing yourself. Instead of randomly piling more things, people and activities into your life, knowing yourself guides you to be selective. Your workouts will be more productive as you are in tune with your body. You'll learn the greatest skill there is to training: autoregulation. Your eating habits will improve for the same reason. It'll even help you know when you've had enough Highland Park and it's time to call it a night (or lunch). Simply put, you will know yourself and will be confident in making decisions when life throws both good, and bad, shit your way. If you are not comfortable with yourself, it's unlikely that anything you read in this book will work for you.

What can you do?

When you train, train. How does the weight feel today? Which muscles are you working when pressing overhead? Is this a day to go heavy or to take it easy?

When you eat, eat. Focus on biting and tasting the food, place the fork down between mouthfuls and check in with yourself and the feelings of fullness. Do I really feel like eating dessert? Does this meal require more ketchup? What's eating Gilbert Grape? When you have dinner with your family or friends, be present and throw your phone somewhere where you can't reach it. Don't always turn on the TV (unless the Stanley Cup playoffs are on).

I guarantee that you will develop a better relationship with not only yourself but also with those close to you. Just because you sit next to someone and eat dinner together doesn't mean that you are close in any way other than physically. Emotionally, you might as well be in Zambia or Switzerland.

Realising that you are doing something while doing it is being mindful. If you scoff down food while checking Facebook, watching the news and YouTubing old *Jackass* highlight reels, and realise it, you are being mindful. You are mindful about what is happening at that very moment. Start small and start inching your way closer to doing a single task at a time. Then, once you've practised in a safe space for a while, and if you are feeling adventurous, you can experiment with masturdating. The king and the queen of all solitude activities. See *A Date with Me (cold night for masturdating)* in the appendix.

I'm risking sounding all spiritual, but what the hell: learning to sit with yourself in solitude is a path to inner peace. And when there's peace within you, it reflects out to your work, relationships and other parts of life. It even helps you to keep calm during the times of unavoidable chaos. The revolution starts by you dangling your arms by your sides. And the revolution will not be televised.

THE VALUE OF MENTAL DELOAD

To have a healthy body requires one to have a healthy mind. You can't have one without the other.

Work – hint: what we do for money – can often take control and priority in life. Whether our aim is to reach a certain paycheck, achieve a specific title or be acknowledged as a leader in our chosen field, life can become out of balance.

I am not saying work is unimportant: it can provide purpose in our days, and financial independence in our lives. But too much work, no matter how meaningful, can throw the rest of our lives out of balance. If we are not careful, our health, both mental and physical, will suffer from bearing the load. We need to balance work and stress with play and discovery. In Western society, rest and relaxation are not valued. Rather, society will applaud you for pursuing a constant hustle and grind.

Yet, for most people, this will eventually lead to some sort of breakdown. I want us to have a more sustainable way of doing things. We need to learn to "deload" while striving for our goals.

Life should be seen as a marathon with built-in rest breaks. It's not done as a sprint. It's common to see people hustling for 20 years while ignoring everything else that life has to offer. They spend 20 years ignoring their health while making money, and then spend the next 20 years spending that money to try and regain their health. Worse yet, they might abuse their body and mind for 20 years and drop dead before there's a chance to enjoy the fruits of their labour.

Learning to play again

Learning to "play" will reinvigorate, de-stress and reignite you. This can improve your odds of achieving your health goals and the body that you want. You will become more present when you are around your family and friends. You will feel calmer and more content and you'll learn to turn off the constant chatter in your head. This will give you breathing room for new ideas. You will feel more productive and creative with your work.

For a few days a week, block time into your schedule for an activity that seemingly doesn't have a means to an end. Pick something that you do only for the sake of that moment. The time block doesn't have to be longer than half an hour. The only rule is to fully immerse yourself in the activity. And it needs to be an activity, not something passive like watching *Seinfeld* or reading about the destruction of ancient civilisations.

A non-comprehensive list of play activities:

- Play an instrument.

- Surf, fly a kite, go mountain biking, hike, do gardening.

- Draw, paint, craft, build the *Starship Enterprise* with Lego. Do something creative with your hands.

If someone saw you doing this activity, they might think you were "wasting" time. But little do they know the power of play. And by the way, fitness training is not play, it's exercise.

Deload and contemplate life

What's the difference between "deload" and "play", then? Deloading can be something you schedule in your calendar weekly for an hour or so. It's your time to contemplate the depths of meaning. It could be going for a walk or writing down your thoughts without any judgement. In a way, it is similar to play in that that you press pause. You take a step back and reflect on what's going on. It allows you to do a possible course correction, if necessary. I like to do this on most evenings along with my gratitude journal.

After reading the article "You're Too Busy. You Need a 'Shultz Hour'" by David Leonhardt in the *New York Times*, I now also block out one hour every week to sit and contemplate without any distraction. Too often we choose a direction, and speed into that direction without ever stopping to see if where we are going is where we want to be. The deload, or the "Shultz Hour", allows you to check in with yourself.

Re-learning to walk

Walking is one of the best things you can do for your mental deload, and you can start doing it today as long as you own a pair of shoes. Heck, you can probably do this barefoot if you're not winning in the shoe section. Whether it's parking your car in the furthest away space in the car park, taking the stairs instead of the lift or going for a short stroll during your lunch hour doesn't matter. What counts is the cumulative effort that adds up over time.

To me, the physical benefits of walking are just an added bonus. I walk because it brings me clarity of mind and an improved mood. Walking is a great time to think. I can't get my head around why anyone would do this indoors on a treadmill, unless there is thunder, lightning or Mr T's fists falling from the sky. Getting outside gives me what I call "the positive environmental effect". You can even practise walking meditation and stop frequently to notice the sun hitting you with its rays, look at the flowers, smell the birds, etc. Good for the body, good for the mind. Sure beats looking at yourself in the mirror and inhaling the vapours off someone next to you who's sweating like a priest in the liquor store. But that's just me. If you are a social creature, create your wolf pack and walk with others. You can talk stuff through, come up with ideas and have meetings while walking. Or only do it to not be glued to the ever-present electronic devices. The options are endless. And if all else fails, rescue a dog from the pound who relies on your walk for a permit to wee. Not having to clean the carpet soaked with dog pee is a powerful walking motivation in itself.

THE LOST ART OF GRACEFULNESS

grace *n.* smoothness and elegance of movement, form, manner or act

There's something to be said about grace and how it can affect the way you look, feel and how you make others feel around you. When you add gracefulness to your days you will end up with a better and healthier body. Imagine yourself sprinting on a treadmill. How graceful does it look? Would you like to see yourself run on a big screen observed by others? If not, think about how you can run more gracefully. It will not only make you more aware of your running technique but is more likely to keep you injury-free. You don't have to run like Usain Bolt or Merlene Ottey but do the best you can to have an aura of gracefulness in your stride. Otherwise in 10 years you will feel like, well, like you've been running with poor technique for 10 years.

When lifting, perform each movement and each lift with the precision of a scientist mixing a cocktail of dynamite and nitrogen: gracefully. Imagine a row of judges scoring you between one and 10. How graceful is your deadlift? When loading the plates onto a bar or picking a kettle-bell off the ground, are you rounding your back and therefore resembling an old beat-up ape? Or are you moving with a straight spine and baring the look of a royal gorilla on top of the food chain ready to take on the jungle? To all you biologists out there, I know gorillas don't have a straight back. Don't get caught up in the details. Gracefulness throughout your gym career will add longevity to your lifting.

Grace goes beyond movement

Are you graceful in your interactions with other people throughout the day? Treat everyone the same no matter who they are and what their stature in life is. In simple terms, don't be a dickhead. Smile often, even to random people. You might make someone's day. Make people feel good when they see you. But don't be creepy. And stop complaining and blaming other people about everything. What actions can you take to improve the situation instead of waiting for someone else to change? Life's better once you realise that you hold the keys to change in almost every situation. There's a door; use it. Gracefully.

How will you be remembered?

Here's a morbid thought that might work: what do you want people to say about you when you're not around anymore? Will they talk about how you lit up their days or did you suck the energy out of the room? Be the better part of someone's life. That doesn't mean that you have to be over the top or make Jamie Foxx look like a wallflower. But have grace about you and the way you interact. Be on time and respect other people. When someone asks you a question and you don't know the answer, admit it. Don't pull a made-up answer from between your butt cheeks just trying to impress someone. There's a lot of grace and humility in "I don't know". You can always say that you'll look into it for them. People appreciate honesty.

When you win, whether it be a pub quiz or the Olympics (of a pub quiz, can you imagine?), do so with grace and acknowledge those who competed against you. When you lose or make a mistake, gracefully accept it and learn from it. Apologise when necessary. Own it and grow from it. There's always something to be learned, even in a pub quiz. Maybe next time you need to put more effort into studying the geology of the sub-Saharan Africa to beat the reigning champions on table two. You know, near the fireplace. In that case, open a book about sub-Saharan Africa. Gracefully, of course.

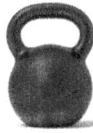

PART 10

This Never Works For Me

THE BORING ANSWERS TO CHALLENGING QUESTIONS

How do I change my eating habits?

In my private coaching group "Rage Against the Calorie Counting" (it's funny, you can laugh), we work together to implement healthier habits over a long period of time. Our simple goal is to make healthy eating second nature. In order to do so, we focus on making healthy eating *reasonable* instead of implementing strict and overbearing rules.

There are a few keystone habits that, when implemented, ingrained and done with consistency, will have a huge impact on your health. (Again, to dive deeper into these habits I recommend Georgie Fear's *Lean Habits* book or the great information provided by Precision Nutrition.)

- Eat mostly wholefoods.

- Eat just enough (so you don't end up too full or still hungry).

- Eat 3–4 serves of protein each day.

↦ Eat a larger amount of vegetables of all colours.

↦ Eat 3–4 meals a day without snacking in between.

None of those are magic solutions, hacks, or tightly guarded secrets. All of these habits are achievable over a period of time, no matter what your starting point.

Yes, some habits will be easy for you to implement and some extremely challenging. It all depends on where you are *right now*. But they are all possible to start and even master without marrying yourself to a new diet or cooking approach.

BEING OPEN TO CHANGE

Someone in the coaching group made an amazing comment, and I wanted to expand on it.

> I just wanted to post a bit of a general note about the habit tracking. I've learnt that you need to be open to change and to trying new things in order to achieve with the habits. For me the hardest thing was breakfast, i was totally stuck on eating my granola, fruit and yogurt for breakfast (or avo on toast!) and didn't really want to change from that. I found it hard to keep full until lunchtime, but was in a habit that i liked. I have recently started making smoothies in the morning (i never thought i would be a smoothie person!) and because of this i can get an extra does of whatever i feel i am missing in the morning, whether that is protein, fruit, peanut butter etc. Now i am completely full until lunch and don't get a 'dip' at 11am. I actually look forward to making my smoothie in the morning and it isn't the chore i thought it would be. This has helped me with a number of the habits so just thought i would share! 😜
>
> Like · Reply · 👍 1 · 1 hr

Eating is a sacred territory for most of us. It's part of our identity. Breaking bread together is how we connect with our loved ones. Dipping fries into mayonnaise is how we turn strangers into friends. Hell, sharing a round of tequila is how some end up sharing a baby nine months later. Changing heavily ingrained eating habits is often a struggle – we might be subconsciously fighting the change.

For these habits to be successfully implemented over the long term, you will have to be willing to change. The motivation behind the change has to be big enough. The option of continuing with your current eating habits has to be more terrifying and morbid than the pain and hardship you'll endure when changing an old, well-ingrained routine to something new. You will have to be willing to step out of what feels natural and into the awkward territory of the unknown. You will have to be willing to change who you are and how you approach eating and your lifestyle in general.

How do I change my training habits?

The information available about fitness training is overwhelming. You can read every post on your favourite blogs. You can read dozens of books. You can hire the best coaches in the world. But all that is useless unless you take action. There's a point when the flood of information becomes paralysing: you're being pulled in 10 different directions at once and end up doing nothing at all. You know what I mean here: "I want to run a marathon", "lose fat", "get stronger", "do gymnastics", "master the kettlebells", "own the Olympic lifts", "tackle the *Battle of Waterloo*-themed obstacle course"... you have too many things to choose from.

Having so many options will leave you feeling lost and unfocused. To make extraordinary progress at anything, you have to pursue one goal relentlessly. Regardless of the goal you have in mind, ask yourself: "Is this what I really want?" If it is, don't worry about other doors closing, for now. If it is not what you really want, well, scrap it. Notice the important part of the question: "I want". It's not "you want", "they want" or "my mum's friend wants". It's "I". Pursue what you really want.

Does this mean that you will be satisfied and driven doing the same thing for the rest of your days? Absolutely not. Let's be honest here. Some decisions are terrible in hindsight, horrendous even. After traveling along a certain path for a while, you might realise that you've been on the wrong road, heading in the wrong direction. You might realise this at a point when it is extremely difficult to change course. It might even feel impossible.

But if you've sincerely pursued a goal that was once important to you, and later changed your mind, there's no shame in that. You went after what felt important, at the time. Sometimes you have to make a decision and choose a goal to chase. Yes, do your research and weigh all the options before deciding. But don't let overthinking paralyse you and prevent you from taking action. Choose one goal and get after it. Otherwise, life will pass you by while you are thinking about all of the options. Before you realise it, you'll be 90 years old and bitter about the safe choices you've made. Don't be afraid to make mistakes. Mistakes mean that you went for it.

KEEP YOUR FOCUS ON WHAT'S IMPORTANT

Keeping your focus on one goal might be the hardest thing to do. To successfully focus on one goal means that you will have to ignore the other 100 goals that everyone else is pursuing. You will feel as if you are going to miss out. A few years back, my goal was to improve my Jefferson deadlift. My training for it was simple: deadlift and press three days a week, that's it. At the end of each session, my mind wandered: "I should do more single leg stuff, carries and conditioning". So I made a deal with myself: to follow the program to the T for six weeks. After that, I can do whatever I want again. If I start adding more "stuff", it's not "the program" – it becomes "the program and stuff". And once that happens, it's hard to judge the success of the program because I added too much "stuff" to it.

Even if you follow the wrong program for a while, it's not the end of the world. It's only training. But if you never experiment or get out of your comfort zone, you'll end up like most people in gyms, doing the same thing over and over and over again. You know the type: a guy or a girl who's looked and felt the same or had the same strength levels for years. Or even worse, he or she keeps doing the same thing, always pushing heavy and getting injured. Or the person who always does the same aerobic classes because it's fun, but she or he has not improved their fitness for five years, because they refuse to try a different approach.

STAY FOCUSED BY FOLLOWING THE PROCESS

1. Choose ONE goal.

2. Choose ONE program that supports that goal.

3. Direct all your focus onto that ONE program.

4. Follow through and finish the program you chose. (This step is surprisingly hard for many.)

5. Re-evaluate. Was it the right goal for you? Did you do well? How could you do better? Do you want to continue pursuing this goal? Is it what you want?

6. Either continue, or choose another goal.

Putting your head down and getting on with it beats eternal contemplation.

Why do my results never last?

Once we decide that we want something, we usually want it *now*. Not tomorrow or 10 weeks from now but *now*, dammit. The issue with *now* is that we are seeking instant gratification and it clouds our rational thinking. We end up focusing on the short-term solution.

Take buying a new piece of clothing for example. You see something hip hanging on the rack at the local store and your brain goes into overdrive. Flashing disco lights come on and the brain chants *buy, buy, buy.* As the chanting gets louder and the lights get brighter you forget the amount of money you have, the gas bill you have to pay tomorrow and the wedding anniversary present you have to buy next month. All you can hear is: "I need to buy this wool sweater because it feels amazing and will make me look like a smooth criminal who should be locked up in the velvety institution of dangerously sexified personnel". All you care about is the instant gratification of owning something new. You forget the long-term effects of having less money for bills, and possibly a looming divorce since you can't afford that anniversary present. You have to fight the buying urge and reason with yourself to walk away from the store empty-handed. Sometimes you won't even be aware of any of this happening in your skull space. Like Nicolaus Copernicus might've said, "Wow. I was not aware of that."

(I know what you are thinking right now. You wanted to read about improving your body and all I do is talk about sweaters and skull space, while misquoting Nicolaus Copernicus. Is nothing sacred anymore!?)

Let me throw some more stardust on your face.

THE ISSUE WITH INSTANT GRATIFICATION

Let's say you see a video clip of Eddie Van Halen shredding a 5-minute brain-melting solo on YouTube and get infected by the guitar-fever bug. You take your infection to the local guitar store and fork out the dough for the devilishly good-looking instrument that is the EVH Wolfgang. Good for you. Since your goal is to become the next bare-chested, leather-pants-wearing guitar hero, you wouldn't place the guitar in the corner of the living room, only to pick it up once a week. No matter how much you paid for the guitar, you can't dust it off just once a week and expect to produce flaming licks in 12 weeks' time. Hell no. On the flip side, if you are a mere mortal, you don't buy the "Five Weeks to Shredding Like Father Eddie" program online, which requires you to play six hours a day. You, a mere mortal, don't have the privilege to sacrifice work, family and other aspects of your daily life. It's just not a reasonable plan for an average person like you or me.

Unless you have some form of hidden virtuoso in you, it would be expected that you practise often and build your playing skills step-by-step over a very long time. To get better at playing, you can't just wish to be better while watching other people playing on Instagram. You have to actually practise and improve your skills, usually in a very tedious way. It will make your fingers and brain hurt. And unless you are willing to sacrifice work, family and other aspects of your life (like bleeding fingers), it's safe to say that you will never play like Father Eddie. You will definitely get better at it over time by improving your skills. But your improvement and long-term guitar playing success is strictly correlated with the amount of time and effort you put in to build your skills.

Similarly, you can't play hardcore for five weeks straight, then not pick up the guitar for a month and expect to have retained all the skills you gained when you first started. No, a little over a long haul makes perfect sense.

You right now: "WTF, Joonas. Enough with the guitars and leather pants and Eddie Van Halen!"

OK, let me pull this all back together for you.

THE ISSUE WITH SHORT-TERM TRANSFORMATIONS

The situation with guitar skills is hard to argue with. For some reason, though, we don't have the same reality filter when viewing our health and fitness goals. We see amazing transformations achieved in the short term, with oiled-up bodies, perky butt cheeks and sculpted chesticles, and we don't think twice about striving for the same. We ignore the facts that are stacked against us. One of them is that we don't have the skills, the time or the resources to put in the effort those bodies require. We are not willing to sacrifice our precious Sunday morning family time, cocktails with friends, or to say no to the Sunday cheesecake. And rightfully so: what's life without cheesecake, anyway? Yet we ignore the obvious and sign up for the "Lounge to a Lean Mofo in 5 weeks" challenge in flocks.

These challenges give us a strict meal plan to follow combined with a hardcore training program, which is always high in intensity and volume. Because let's be honest, making people tired is a cheap way to provide the illusion of a great workout. No wonder the participants lose weight. I mean, eating limited calories and training for the zombie apocalypse will do that for you.

When we see amazing transformations achieved in a short time we choose (because we know the true answer) to ignore what happens once the initial transformation period is over. We follow a strict plan that works in the perfect life. Yet with this plan, everything is given to us on a platter and we don't have to learn the skills necessary for when life gets complicated. It might feel great at the time but we don't know how to adjust our habits to match our busy schedules once the program is over. We, unlike Nicolaus Copernicus, don't know what we don't know.

THE SKILL DEFICIT

Like with anything that you want to achieve and improve at, you need to work on your healthy eating and training skills. What happens when you can only train 20 minutes a day, twice a week? What happens when you don't have time to count calories and portion your meals into Tupperware containers each Sunday? Or when your boss asks you out for lunch and doesn't appreciate your suggestion of sitting on the park bench while you dig into your containers of steamed green beans and lightly salted ocean perch? Short-term plans don't teach you the skills you need to be successful with your health and fitness for the rest of your life.

The more skills you have in a certain area, the more flexibility you have to "wing it", to modify things on the fly. If you don't have the skills, you can't expect to improvise and adjust. You will always be the one who follows other people's plans. And no matter how exceptional their plans are, they're never yours.

I am not saying that strict short-term transformations are worthless. As long as you are not a beginner to training and healthy eating, prone to body-image issues or orthorexic eating, these can be great challenges to get ready for an event. But it shouldn't be anyone's entry point into training and fitness. If you don't have the skills, the results won't last. Over time, you might end up in a worse position than when you first started. Most of us shouldn't focus on where we'll be in five weeks, but where we'll be in 10 years. And that's why *reasonable* done with consistency beats *extreme* done periodically.

INSTEAD OF ADDING MORE, TRY ELIMINATING

What usually happens when we get stuck and we stop progressing towards our health and training goals? We either try to train more often or eat more strictly in whatever way has brought us some success in the past. There is nothing wrong with this approach, if it works. But more of the same is not always the answer. It's helpful to take a step back to analyse why you aren't having any success or why you stopped doing what worked in the past. What got you side-tracked or what stopped you from getting on track in the first place?

What if you could take the opposite approach and, instead of adding more, simply eliminate anything that's unnecessary? You might find what's truly holding you back and get to the core of the problem instead of just piling more "solutions" on top of an already non-functioning foundation. Think of it as building a skyscraper; how often do you think the engineers say, "Well, we haven't really stabilised the foundation and the basement is flooding, but let's see if we can fix it by adding a penthouse and an antenna"? I mean, I'm not an engineer and I've built very few skyscrapers in my time (read: none), but to me, it doesn't make any sense.

What if, instead, you found one core issue holding you back? If you could eliminate one thing, habit, situation or even a person (as in, limit your time with the person, not like really "eliminate" them. Because that would be wrong. You'd go to jail for that. And hell. You definitely don't want to go to hell), you might find your way towards exceptional results.

If you always take the same route to work and stop on the way to get a cream cheese bagel from Dougie, try taking a different route. Do you frequently skip your training session after work because you're too tired? Try scheduling your training session first thing in the morning or during lunch hours. If you always eat cookies at work and it happens unintentionally when you go to the break room to refill your tea, come up with a solution that will stop you from going to the break room at all. That way, you won't have to fight with your willpower, as the cookie jar won't be close enough to tempt you in the first place. All those things are reasonably simple to change, even if Dougie is the nicest guy around and his bagels have the creamiest of all cheeses.

What can be challenging, though, is to distance yourself from friends or even family members who might have a negative influence on you. We're talking about the type of person whose very presence leads you to engage in less-than-ideal behaviour. It could even be a person who always makes you feel like crap (intentionally or not), which then results in you making poor decisions to try and comfort yourself. In the age of social media, we all know people who are always complaining about something or feeling sorry for themselves. Block them from your newsfeed. Otherwise, they will subconsciously bring you down, guaranteed. It can be hard to say "no" to such people, but eventually you've got to decide what is essential and what's not.

Before trying to do more of the same, think about what is holding you back and see if it is possible to eliminate or change it. Sometimes it's as simple as taking a different route to work. Or it can be something deeper such as dealing with your past ghosts in order to finally get some traction and move forward. Once you find your obstacles, accept and eliminate them if possible, things will start to move forward faster than you ever thought possible.

FINAL WORDS

For Now

In full disclosure, I don't believe it's possible to ever truly master the balance between health, life and fitness. Having a perfect balance is an illusion which requires multiple factors, some of which are outside of your control, to go your way. So, when you feel like you've finally figured out the perfect balance, it will only be for a fading moment. And that's OK.

Mastery means understanding principles so it's possible to implement them with greater flexibility as life happens. Not breaking and letting go, but bending to make the principles work in whatever life throws your way. At times it can feel like an endless, frustrating struggle. But as with any other skill, the more you practise, the closer to mastery you'll get.

Use these principles and let them flex and morph depending on what's going on in your life at any given time. Aim higher when possible. Know when to take it easier. Then steer back to the middle and reassess.

It's not the most exciting advice, but it's the one that works.

WHAT'S NEXT?

A while from now, once you've implemented the principles and steps in this book, email me at **joonas@repsandtherest.com**, or leave a review on Amazon. I can't wait to hear about your success and all the amazing things you've done with your newly found strength, fitness and confidence.

P.S. If you happen to be Elon Musk and these principles help you to manage your health and fitness while you are busy colonising Mars, I'd love to hear about that too. Also, if it's not too much to ask, could you name one of your big rockets *No Spandex on Combustion*. Just a thought, it's not like I'm forcing you to do it.

FURTHER READING

My knowledge is the product of the people that I've learned from. Health and fitness ideas are rarely novel or new. I don't know if anything I've written in this book is ground-breaking. More likely, it is a combination of ideas I've learned from others by either reading their books or listening to them graciously share their knowledge. All I can hope is that I've added my own twisted and distorted angle to further expand and open these ideas to a new audience. The following authors and their books are the originals, for me, anyway.

ON FITNESS...

Dan John, *Never Let Go* (start with it, then read all his other books)
I got my introduction to reasonable fitness through Dan John's writing. His written wisdom changed it for me, and I am forever grateful.

Michael Boyle, *New Functional Training for Sports (2nd Edition)*
I am often just a cook modifying Mike Boyle's recipes.

Bill Hartman, *All Gain, No Pain*
The plan in here isn't watered down to appeal for the masses. Much more than just a training program.

ON HEALTH...

Georgie Fear, *Lean Habits*
The nutrition habits in here could be all you'll ever need.

Frank Forencich, *The Art is Long*
If we want to live a long and healthy life, and allow future generations to do the same, we need to do more. This is the next step.

Bhante Gunaratana, *Mindfulness in Plain English*
Meditating will help you to slow down. And no, you don't need to believe in anything supernatural to do it.

Charles Duhigg, *The Power of Habit*
The habit loop. Understanding it makes changing, removing and adding habits easier.

ON LIFE...

Brené Brown, *Daring Greatly*
Her books and research hit home for me, hard.

Greg McKeown, *Essentialism*
Many books have been written about prioritising time. This one is my favourite.

Patti Smith, *M Train*
Coffee, art and everything in-between.

For more book recommendations, go to **RepsAndTheRest.com**

ACKNOWLEDGEMENTS

Writing is hard. And although the typing itself is mostly a solo effort, there are many pieces that go into putting together a book. I'd like to thank the following people for helping me piece together this book.

Pat Flynn (ChroniclesOfStrength.com), for giving me much-needed guidance when I was struggling with the editing of this book.

Dan John, the original title for this book was *Reasonable Fitness*, an idea I got from Dan's writing. Not only was he kind enough to let me use it, he sent me an avalanche of his articles to support the topic.

All my teachers (whether I've met you or not) and colleagues, past and present, who have shaped my understanding of health and fitness to what it is today. I hope I can have at least a fraction of the positive impact on others that you've had on me.

All my clients, past and present, for trusting me with your health and fitness. I truly believe that I have one of the best jobs in the world because of you. And I try hard to never take any of it for granted.

Chris Vein, for embracing "the gospel of Joonas" with your foreword. You do know how to write after all! By the way, you got "your life back" because of your drive to do it. I only gave you directions, you made it happen.

Bec Sharp, for being the cheerleader of my writing, especially during the early stages of my blog. I really needed it. Thank you!

My editor, Jessica Hoadley, for taking my non-linear and at times painfully rambling manuscript and editing it into a book I could be proud of. You did it without ever losing the authentic sound of me. What a difference you made. Thank you.

Stephanie Bruckner, for providing honest feedback in the early stages of the writing. See those Q and A lines in various chapters? That's you.

Michal Palus, for asking "why" with everything I did. It made this book so much better. But dammit, it was annoying at the time.

Mum and Dad, for encouraging me to write, and for showing me by example what lifelong health is all about. I know, it took me a while to listen on both. Kiitos.

And Colleen, for putting up with my, at times, moody self while trying to figure out this book. Thank you for everything that we have. With you I smile wider and laugh harder.

APPENDIX 1

A Date Night with Me
(a cold night for masturdating)

A few years back I spent a cold winter weekend in Newcastle, about 150 km north of Sydney where I was doing a course with the Postural Restoration Institute. After we finished on Saturday afternoon I had the night in the city by all myself. I was free to roam the streets of a small town. And, as any man with a lot of time on his hands would do, I organized a date, with Me.

This is a true and unedited recollection of that night. Back in the day before I adopted a "mostly plant-based diet".

THE DAY BEFORE

The evening before, I was scratching my head trying to figure out where should I take Me on a date? After looking through different options on Google I found a nice craft beer bar serving hearty meals right around the corner from where I was staying. I knew that this place would wow Me over. It was a given, knowing Me's enthusiasm for craft beers and appreciation for thick-cut chips. It didn't hurt that the bar was dimly lit and oozed a twisted baroque character, creating the perfect environment for a romantic date. This would be perfect.

I promised Me not to bury my head in the menu, not to check my phone and not to bring a book. I also promised Me not to rewind the just-finished day in my head and not to let tomorrow's second day of the course consume my thoughts. In other words, I promised Me to be completely present in the moment, no matter how awkward things might get. I would put all my focus on Me, the meal, the beer and the atmosphere.

I even decided to wear a reasonably casual outfit, to not seem too desperate to please Me with my sense of fashion. Me should like my style as it is, I thought.

DATE NIGHT – 7 PM

I left the hostel (what can I say, I am a big spender) early as the rain was mounting up, jogging across the park to avoid getting soaked before the date. I had agreed to meet Me at the bar at 7 pm and, punctual Scandinavian that I am, arrived a few minutes early just to be sure I wouldn't be late. Nothing worse than keeping someone waiting. By the time I arrived, the bar was already filling up and a hint of worry drifted through me: would there be room for Me?

But, seasoned bar-penguin that I am, I swayed my way through the crowds and arrived at the bar counter just in time to meet Me. We shook hands and it lead into an elaborate exchange of various forms of fist pumps. As I was reading through the beer selection I exchanged a few quick words with the tired-looking bartender and decided to go with Mornington Peninsula Brewery's porter. If there's a highway to melt Me's heart it's a strong porter that packs a punch, and this one didn't disappoint. Off to a great start, I thought to myself as the first drops of porter flowed through my lips.

With my Arctic hawk eyes looking for empty seats, I was weighing up the options in my head. The mission at hand required privacy, so sharing a table with others would be out of the question. I kept looking around until my eyes locked on the empty stools and high table in the middle of the room. Just enough privacy without looking like I wanted to hide Me in the dark corners of the room, like some sort of dismembered creature that couldn't stand to be in plain sight. No, I wanted everyone to know that I was proud to be dating Me that night.

DATE NIGHT — 7.15 PM

As I sat down, my level of hunger was seemingly uncontrollable. I was afraid I would blow' the negative fuse on the date. Due to the hectic schedule of the day so far, my eating habits had required some flexibility and I hadn't had anything that resembled food since 1 pm. At that time I still had a bad track record of making poor meal choices when in a ravenous state of hunger. I was anxious that I would settle for a meal that wouldn't be delicious enough. I was afraid that the hunger would cloud my judgement of the menu, ruining the date. I started to feel pearls of sweat forming on my forehead. My tongue was starting to shake causing unnecessarily loud slurping sounds while bouncing between the lower and upper teeth.

The pressure was fuming through my now already semi-closed and tired eyelids. This was the make-or-break moment of the date and everything would be judged by this one decision – what meal do I order for Me?

After tossing between the rib eye and the sirloin I decided to go with the 250 gm Angus beef sirloin cooked medium-rare, served with charred corn, thick fries, slaw and porter jus. I opted for extra-smoky barbeque sauce on the side. Thick-cut chips required the sauce, that much was certain. Satisfied with my decision-making skills in a high-pressure situation, I relaxed onto the stool and nursed the beer with a new-found enthusiasm.

DATE NIGHT – 7.25 PM

To take my mind off my hunger I ordered another beer, Murray's Craft Brewing Co's Dark Knight porter. Safe choice, I thought, but why risk it when the night so far had been a success. Why ruin it all and try to be adventurous by ordering something like an always-disappointing wheat beer. Besides, I was hungry. If there is one thing I know, it's that when you are carrying a canister of aviation fuel, you don't want to play with the engines. Especially while trying to please Me.

So I sunk back onto my stool, had a small sip of the beer, swirled it in my mouth and appreciated the fact that I was inside, drinking beer, had food on the way and was sheltered from the thunderous rain of the outside world. There was no obsessing over my phone or worries that I'd have to pick a newspaper to read just to look busy. None of it. I was having good time with Me. And despite the noise of the crowd around Me, my head was silent.

DATE NIGHT – 7.45 PM

The meal arrived, and all my worries were whisked away. The dead piece of cow lying on the plate in front of me was cooked to perfection. The pile of chips was towering, so I wouldn't have to return to the hotel via a convenience store. The salad was crispy and the only way the barbeque sauce could've been smokier was to have an actual campfire burning next to it.

I took my time with the meal, focusing on chewing each mouthful and placing the fork on the plate between each helping so I could feel the grinding of food between my teeth. I sipped the beer with patience, unheard of in the brief history of my existence. But what made the situation meaningful was that I was giving all my attention to Me. I didn't let anything or anyone be a distraction. This was a Zen-version of *Saturday Night Fever.* I was John Travolta without the moves, the outfit or the fever.

DATE NIGHT – 8.20 PM

But all the good things must come to an end. After two tasty porters, a great cow and a heavy dose of barbeque sauce, I was ready to call it a night and take Me back to my hotel. After all, I would have to be sharp for the next day and ordering another porter would steer my determination off course. No matter how good the company of Me was. I got up, thanked the bartender on my way out and walked into a cold and rainy Newcastle night with Me. The long overdue date night had been a success.

Why does any of this matter? Why should you care about masturdating?

It all starts with you. I tend to live in my head, working on something that will make me feel that I am striving forward, all the time. Whether it's studying, reading, writing, or whatever, I find it hard to "switch off" and chill without the thought of *not* accomplishing something. So if you recognise yourself as a Type A, someone who is always on, or just someone who doesn't know how to be on their own, look at your calendar and book a date with Me. Make it special and Me will appreciate it.

Learning to sit in peace with yourself will help your relationships with others as well. If you can't be content and live in the moment when spending time by yourself, how can you be content with anyone or anything else?

I got the idea for masturdating after reading a great blog post by Nate Green on NateGreen.org.

APPENDIX 2

Blank Training Program Templates

SESSION A: Reset and Movement Preparation			
Movement	Sets	Repetitions	Your Notes
9090 Breathing with a Hip Lift	1-2	4 Breaths	
Quadruped Breathing	1-2	4 Breaths	
Scapula, Shoulder, Hip CARS	1	3 each way	
Tactical Frog	1	10	
Downward Dog to Step to Rotation	1	2 each side	
Glute Hip Lift	1	5 each leg	
Squat to Stand	1	5	
Standing Cross Crawl	1	5 each side	
Farmer Carry	1	60 seconds	

Phase 1, Session A	Day 1	Day 2	Day 3	Day 4

Power and Resistance Training	weight x reps x sets	weight x reps x sets	weight x reps x sets	weight x reps x sets
A1	x8x2	x8x3	x10x2	x10x3
A2	x8x2	x8x3	x10x2	x10x3
B1	x8x2	x8x3	x10x2	x10x3
B2	x8x2	x8x3	x10x2	x10x3
B3	3-4 breaths x2	3-4 breaths x3	4-5 breaths x2	4-5 breaths x3

Conditioning	Day 1	Day 2	Day 3	Day 4

SESSION B: Reset and Movement Preparation			
Movement	Sets	Repetitions	Your Notes
9090 Breathing with a Hip Lift	1-2	4 Breaths	
Quadruped Breathing	1-2	4 Breaths	
Scapula, Shoulder, Hip CARS	1	3 each way	
Tactical Frog	1	10	
Downward Dog to Step to Rotation	1	2 each side	
Glute Hip Lift	1	5 each leg	
Squat to Stand	1	5	
Standing Cross Crawl	1	5 each side	
Suitcase Carry	1	30 seconds/hand	

Phase 1, Session B	Day 1	Day 2	Day 3	Day 4

Power and Resistance Training	weight x reps x sets	weight x reps x sets	weight x reps x sets	weight x reps x sets
A1	x8x2	x8x3	x10x2	x10x3
A2	x8x2	x8x3	x10x2	x10x3
B1	x8x2	x8x3	x10x2	x10x3
B2	x8x2	x8x3	x10x2	x10x3
B3	3-4 breaths x2	3-4 breaths x3	4-5 breaths x2	4-5 breaths x3

Conditioning	Session 1	Session 2	Session 3	Session 4

SESSION A: Reset and Movement Preparation			
Movement	Sets	Repetitions	Your Notes
9090 Breathing with a Hip Lift	1-2	4 Breaths	
Quadruped Breathing	1-2	4 Breaths	
Scapula, Shoulder, Hip CARS	1	3 each way	
Tactical Frog	1	10	
Downward Dog to Step to Rotation	1	2 each side	
Glute Hip Lift	1	5 each leg	
Squat to Stand	1	5	
Standing Cross Crawl	1	5 each side	
Farmer Carry	1	60 seconds	

Phase 2, Session A	Day 1	Day 2	Day 3	Day 4

Power and Resistance Training	weight x reps x sets	weight x reps x sets	weight x reps x sets	weight x reps x sets
A1	x4x2	x4x3	x5x2	x5x3
A2	3-4 breaths x2	3-4 breaths x3	4-5 breaths x2	4-5 breaths x3
B1	x12x2	x12x3	x15x2	x10x3
B2	x12x2	x12x3	x15x2	x10x3
C1	x12x2	x12x3	x15x2	x10x3
C2	x12x2	x12x3	x15x2	x10x3

Conditioning	Day 1	Day 2	Day 3	Day 4

SESSION B: Reset and Movement Preparation			
Movement	Sets	Repetitions	Your Notes
9090 Breathing with a Hip Lift	1-2	4 Breaths	
Quadruped Breathing	1-2	4 Breaths	
Scapula, Shoulder, Hip CARS	1	3 each way	
Tactical Frog	1	10	
Downward Dog to Step to Rotation	1	2 each side	
Glute Hip Lift	1	5 each leg	
Squat to Stand	1	5	
Standing Cross Crawl	1	5 each side	
Suitcase Carry	1	30 seconds/hand	

Phase 2, Session B	Day 1	Day 2	Day 3	Day 4

Power and Resistance Training	weight x reps x sets	weight x reps x sets	weight x reps x sets	weight x reps x sets
A1	x4x2	x4x3	x5x2	x5x3
A2	3-4 breaths x2	3-4 breaths x3	4-5 breaths x2	4-5 breaths x3
B1	x12x2	x12x3	x15x2	x15x3
B2	x12x2	x12x3	x15x2	x15x3
C1	x12x2	x12x3	x15x2	x15x3
C2	x12x2	x12x3	x15x2	x15x3

Conditioning	Session 1	Session 2	Session 3	Session 4

SESSION A: Reset and Movement Preparation			
Movement	Sets	Repetitions	Your Notes
9090 Breathing with a Hip Lift	1-2	4 Breaths	
Quadruped Breathing	1-2	4 Breaths	
Scapula, Shoulder, Hip CARS	1	3 each way	
Tactical Frog	1	10	
Downward Dog to Step to Rotation	1	2 each side	
Glute Hip Lift	1	5 each leg	
Squat to Stand	1	5	
Standing Cross Crawl	1	5 each side	
Farmer Carry	1	60 seconds	

Phase 3, Session A	Day 1	Day 2	Day 3	Day 4

Power and Resistance Training	weight x reps x sets	weight x reps x sets	weight x reps x sets	weight x reps x sets
A1	x4x3	x5x3	x4x3	x4x4
A2	3-4 breaths x3	4-5 breaths x3	5-6 breaths x2	5-6 breaths x3
B1	x8x3	x10x3	x8x4	x10x4
B2	x8x3	x10x3	x8x4	x10x4
C1	x8x3	x10x3	x8x4	x10x4
C2	x8x3	x10x3	x8x4	x10x4

Conditioning	Day 1	Day 2	Day 3	Day 4

SESSION B: Reset and Movement Preparation			
Movement	Sets	Repetitions	Your Notes
9090 Breathing with a Hip Lift	1-2	4 Breaths	
Quadruped Breathing	1-2	4 Breaths	
Scapula, Shoulder, Hip CARS	1	3 each way	
Tactical Frog	1	10	
Downward Dog to Step to Rotation	1	2 each side	
Glute Hip Lift	1	5 each leg	
Squat to Stand	1	5	
Standing Cross Crawl	1	5 each side	
Suitcase Carry	1	30 seconds/hand	

Phase 3, Session B	Day 1	Day 2	Day 3	Day 4

Power and Resistance Training	weight x reps x sets	weight x reps x sets	weight x reps x sets	weight x reps x sets
A1	x3x2	x3x3	x4x3	x5x3
A2	3-4 breaths x3	4-5 breaths x3	5-6 breaths x2	5-6 breaths x3
B1	x8x3	x10x3	x8x4	x10x4
B2	x12x2	x12x3	x15x2	x15x3
C1	x12x2	x12x3	x15x2	x15x3
C2	x12x2	x12x3	x15x2	x15x3

Conditioning	Session 1	Session 2	Session 3	Session 4

ABOUT THE AUTHOR

Joonas Heikkinen is a personal trainer who works with everyday people struggling with strength, fitness and confidence after being injured. A former fitness addict, he now teaches people how to get and keep results using a *reasonable* approach to fitness.

Growing up in the harsh Arctic temperatures of Finland explains Joonas' deep affection for black coffee, heavy metal and the eternal search for sunshine. In his spare time, he embraces the reasonable approach to playing the guitar and learning improv theatre. His imminent future focus is the less-reasonable approach to learning how to change nappies. He lives in Sydney, Australia, with his wife Colleen.

RepsAndTheRest.com

www.ingramcontent.com/pod-product-compliance
Lightning Source LLC
Chambersburg PA
CBHW072123020426
42334CB00018B/1690